Diagnosis and Management of Parkinson's Disease

First Edition

Cheryl H. Waters, MD

Associate Professor of Medicine
Department of Neurology
University of Southern California
Los Angeles, California

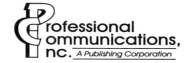
Professional
Communications,
Inc. *A Publishing Corporation*

Published by:
Professional Communications, Inc.

For orders only, please call:
1-800-337-9838

ISBN: 1-884735-33-9

Printed in the United States of America

This text is printed on recycled paper.

DEDICATION

This book is dedicated to my supportive husband, Paul; my four wonderful children, Stephanie, Richard, Jesse and Sam; and, my brave and devoted patients.

ACKNOWLEDGMENT

I would like to acknowledge the support and efforts of the National Parkinson Foundation.

TABLE OF CONTENTS

Definition and Classification	**1**
Epidemiology	**2**
Natural History	**3**
Etiology	**4**
Pathogenesis	**5**
Pathophysiology	**6**
Diagnosis	**7**
Treatment	**8**
Complications of Parkinson's Disease and Its Therapy	**9**
Nonpharmacologic Management of Parkinson's Disease	**10**
Surgery	**11**
Index	**12**

TABLES

Table 1.1   Classification of Parkinsonism 12

Table 7.1   Motor and Nonmotor Symptoms of
Parkinson's Disease 59

Table 7.2   Comparison of Parkinson's Disease and
Essential Tremor 61

Table 7.3   Comparison of Parkinson's and
Parkinson-Plus Diseases 65

Table 7.4   Neuroleptics and Related Agents 67

Table 7.5   Miscellaneous Drugs Associated
With Parkinsonism 68

Table 7.6   Differential Diagnosis of Drug-Induced
Parkinsonism and Parkinson's Disease 69

Table 7.7   Unified Rating Scale for Parkinsonism 74

Table 7.8   Step-Second Test 82

Table 7.9   Schwab and England Activities of
Daily Living Scale 83

Table 8.1   Antiparkinson Agents 91

Table 8.2   Ascending Dosage Schedule for
Pramipexole (Mirapex) 110

Table 8.3   Ascending Dosage Schedule for
Ropinirole (Requip) 115

Table 8.4   COMT Inhibitors 126

Table 9.1   Possible Mechanisms of Levodopa-Related
Motor Fluctuations 142

Table 9.2   Treatment of Motor Complications of
Parkinson's Disease 146

Table 9.3   Presentation Patterns of Levodopa-Related
Dyskinesias Among 168 Patients 152

Table 9.4   Treatment of Behavioral/Psychiatric
Disorders Associated With
Parkinson's Disease 155

Table 10.1   Topics for Discussion Early in Course of
Parkinson's Disease 170

Table 10.2   Selected Patient Education
Materials and Sources 174

| Table 10.3 | Exercises to Relieve Rigidity and Bradykinesia | 179 |

| Table 10.4 | Occupations and Age at Diagnosis of Authors With Parkinson's Disease | 182 |

| Table 10.5 | Parkinson's Disease Foundations | 186 |

| Table 11.1 | Complications Related to Chronic Thalamic Stimulation | 203 |

| Table 11.2 | Published Outcomes of Fetal Transplantation | 209 |

FIGURES

| Figure 3.1 | The Progressive Changes in Parkinson's Disease | 20 |

| Figure 4.1 | Subregional Divisions of the Pars Compacta of the Substantia Nigra | 25 |

| Figure 4.2 | Comparisons of Age- and Parkinson's Disease-Related Nigrostrial Neuron Loss | 26 |

| Figure 5.1 | The Basal Ganglia | 32 |

| Figure 5.2 | The Normal Substantia Nigra | 33 |

| Figure 5.3 | Major Anatomic Pathways To and Within the Basal Ganglia | 34 |

| Figure 5.4 | Neurotransmitter Balance in Normal and Dopamine-Depleted Brain | 37 |

| Figure 5.5 | The Dopaminergic Neuron | 39 |

| Figure 5.6 | The Parkinson Lesion | 42 |

| Figure 5.7 | The Lewy Body | 43 |

| Figure 7.1 | Essential Tremor | 60 |

| Figure 8.1 | Therapeutic Algorithm for Management of Parkinson's Disease | 89 |

| Figure 8.2 | Comparative Mortality in Patients Treated With Levodopa Alone and With Levodopa and Selegiline | 100 |

| Figure 8.3 | "Off" Periods Associated With Pramipexole and Placebo | 108 |

| Figure 8.4 | Ropinirole vs. Levodopa in Early Disease of UPDRS Motor Score | 112 |

Figure 8.5   Ropinirole and Bromocriptine as
             Monotherapy: Comparative Improvement
             in UPDRS Motor Score 113

Figure 8.6   Ropinirole and Placebo: 12-Month
             UPDRS and CGI Results 114

Figure 8.7   Mean "Off" and "On" Times With
             and Without Dyskinesia:
             Tolcapone and Placebo 118

Figure 8.8   Efficacy of Tolcapone After 12 Months 121

Figure 8.9   Plasma Levodopa Concentrations During
             Adjunctive Entacapone 123

Figure 8.10 Effect of Entacapone on
             Daily Total "On" Time 124

Figure 9.1   Efficacy of Levodopa With
             Continuing Treatment 144

Figure 9.2   Development of Levodopa-Related
             Motor Fluctuations 145

Figure 9.3   The "Wearing-Off" Response 147

Figure 9.4   Spectrum of "Off" State Symptoms 148

Figure 10.1 Selected Exercises With Verbal Cues for
             the Parkinson's Disease Patient 175

Figure 11.1 Patterns of Neural Activity Within
             the Basal Ganglia 193

Figure 11.2 Basal Ganglia Circuitry 195

Figure 11.3 Change in Parkinsonian Tremor With
             Chronic Thalamic Stimulation 202

Introduction

The clinical management of the 1 million Americans afflicted with Parkinson's disease is poised to undergo major changes based on recent advances in pharmacologic and surgical therapy that promise significant improvement in patients' quality of life. Many of the new products and procedures are already available and others are in development or clinical trial. Among them are:

- A range of new and novel dopamine agonists
- Methods of altering the administration, delivery, absorption, and metabolism of levodopa
- The possibility of neuroprotective therapy
- The potential manipulation of other neurotransmitter systems
- Novel surgical therapies
- New molecular biological neuroconstructive procedures and operative techniques that use gene therapy.

Thus, the future looks optimistic for the maintenance of Parkinson's disease patients within the mainstream despite the continuing search for cause and cure of the disease.

The Diagnosis and Management of Parkinson's Disease has been prepared for physicians as a review of the etiology, pathophysiology, differential diagnosis, treatment, and management of Parkinson's disease. The author wishes to thank the investigators and clinicians whose experience and publications have supplemented her own as an investigator for the new pharmacologic therapies and made possible this up-to-date presentation of their applicability, efficacy, and nuances.

— *Cheryl H. Waters, MD*

1 Definition and Classification

Parkinson's disease (PD) is the most prevalent type of parkinsonism, a clinical syndrome caused by lesions in the basal ganglia, predominantly in the substantia nigra, that produce deficits in motor behavior.

Parkinsonism is a clinical rather than an etiologic entity since it is associated with several pathologic processes that damage the extrapyramidal system. Its many causes are divided into four categories (Table 1.1):

- Primary, or idiopathic (PD)
- Secondary parkinsonism (associated with infectious agents, drugs, toxins, vascular disease, trauma, brain neoplasm)
- Parkinson-plus syndromes
- Heredodegenerative diseases.

Parkinson's Disease

Parkinson's disease makes up approximately 80% of cases of parkinsonism.[1] The syndrome was first cogently described by James Parkinson in 1817 and named paralysis agitans by Marshall Hall in 1841.[2] Both description and label stress reduction in muscle power unduly, however, omitting rigidity and slowness of movement (akinesia), crucial to the characteristic tetrad known as TRAP:

- Resting **T**remor
- Cogwheel **R**igidity
- Bradykinesia/**A**kinesia
- **P**ostural reflex impairment.

Of this tetrad, only resting tremor is truly suggestive of PD, an early sign that may remain prominent

TABLE 1.1 — CLASSIFICATION OF PARKINSONISM

Idiopathic Parkinsonism
- Parkinson's disease

Secondary Parkinsonism
- Drug-induced
  - Dopamine receptor blockers (neuroleptics)
  - Dopamine depleters (reserpine, tetrabenazine)
  - Lithium
  - Flunarizine, cinnarizine, diltiazem
- Hemiatrophy-hemiparkinsonism
- Hydrocephalus
  - Normal pressure hydrocephalus
  - Noncommunicating hydrocephalus
- Hypoxia
- Infectious
  - Fungal infections
  - AIDS
  - Intracytoplasmic hyaline inclusion disease
  - Subacute sclerosing panencephalitis
  - Postencephalitic
  - Creutzfeldt-Jakob disease
- Metabolic
  - Hypocalcemic parkinsonism
  - Chronic hepatocerebral degeneration
- Paraneoplastic parkinsonism
- Psychogenic
- Syringomesencephalia
- Trauma
- Toxin
  - MPTP intoxication
  - Carbon monoxide intoxication
  - Manganese intoxication
  - Cyanide
  - Methanol
  - Carbon disulfide intoxication
  - Disulfiram
- Tumor
- Vascular
  - Multi-infarct
  - Binswanger's disease

Parkinson-Plus Syndromes
- Cortical-basal ganglionic degeneration
- Dementia syndrome
  - Alzheimer's disease
  - Cortical diffuse Lewy body disease
  - Pick's disease
- Lytico-Bodig (Guamanian PD-D-ALS)
- Multiple system atrophy syndromes
  - Striatonigral degeneration
  - Shy-Drager syndrome
  - Sporadic olivopontocerebellar atrophy
  - Motor neuron disease-Parkinson
- Progressive pallidal atrophy
- Progressive supranuclear palsy

Heredodegenerative Diseases
- Ceroid-lipofuscinosis
- Gerstmann-Strausler-Scheinker disease
- Hallervorden-Spatz
- Huntington's disease
- Lubag (Filipino X-linked dystonia-parkinson)
- Machado-Joseph disease
- Mitochondrial cytopathies with striatal necrosis
- Neuroacanthocytosis
- Familial olivopontocerebellar atrophy
- Thalamic dementia syndrome
- Wilson's disease

Abbreviations: AIDS, acquired immune deficiency syndrome; MPTP, 1-methyl-4-phenyl-1,2,3,6-tetrahydropyridine; PD-D-ALS, Parkinson's disease-dementia-amyotrophic lateral sclerosis.

even late in the disorder.[2] The others occur in varying degrees in other forms of parkinsonism.

Secondary Parkinsonism

■ Postencephalitic Parkinsonism

Many patients who survived the acute febrile illness and encephalopathy during the 1919-to-1926 pandemics of encephalitis lethargica (von Economo's encephalitis) later developed a variety of movement disorders, including parkinsonism.[1] Although the virus(es) that caused the disease was never isolated, parkinsonism is associated with Coxsackie, Japanese B, and western equine encephalitis viruses. The underlying lesion in postencephalitic parkinsonism, depletion of the pigmented, dopamine-secreting neurons in an area of the substantia nigra, is similar to that of PD, but the former has a long latency after exposure to acute illness (a phenomenon not yet understood).

■ Drug-Induced Parkinsonism

A syndrome clinically indistinguishable from PD can be caused by drugs that:

- Deplete the synaptic stores of dopamine (reserpine)
- Block the dopamine receptors (antipsychotics and antiemetics)
- Cause selective destruction of the dopamine nigrostriatal pathway (the street drug contaminant methylphenyltetrahydropyridine [MPTP]).

The parkinsonian syndrome caused by these drugs is often clinically indistinguishable from PD.

■ Pugilistic Encephalopathy

Although some studies suggest that patients with PD may have had a higher incidence of significant head injuries with loss of consciousness than matched controls, others argue against the causative role of trauma.[3,4]

The widespread neurological dysfunction seen in the chronic traumatic encephalopathy of "punch drunk" boxers may include some signs and symptoms of advanced PD, such as:

- Personality changes
- Memory impairment

- Dysarthria
- Tremor
- Ataxia.[3]

This "pugilistic dementia", unlike PD, is caused by severe blows to the brain stem and rotational torques, probably resulting in a series of microhemorrhages.

Parkinson-Plus

Patients with Parkinson-plus carry other features not associated with PD, including:[1]
- Supranuclear gaze palsy (progressive supranuclear palsy)
- Dysautonomia (multiple system atrophy, Shy-Drager syndrome)
- Laryngeal stridor (striatonigral degeneration)
- Apraxia, myoclonus, and alien hand (corticobasal ganglionic degeneration)
- Dementia syndrome (Alzheimer's disease, Lewy body disease)
- Amyotrophic lateral sclerosis (Lytico-Bodig, Guamanian Parkinson's disease-dementia-amyotrophic lateral sclerosis [PD-D-ALS]).

Heredodegenerative Parkinsonism

Inherited degenerative disorders include:
- Wilson's disease (a disease of copper metabolism)
- Huntington's disease
- Hallervorden-Spatz disease, manifest by childhood- or adult-onset progressive dementia, bradykinesia, rigidity, and spasticity, as well as other signs of basal ganglionic degeneration
- Familial basal ganglia calcification
- Familial olivopontocerebellar atrophy.

REFERENCES

1. Jankovic J. The extrapyramidal disorders. In: Bennett JC, Plum F, eds. *Cecil Textbook of Medicine.* 20th ed. Philadelphia, Pa: WB Saunders Co; 1996:2042-2046.

2. Adams RD, Victor M, Ropper AH. *Principles of Neurology.* 6th ed. New York, NY: McGraw-Hill; 1997:1067-1078.

3. Goetz CG, Jankovic J, Koller WC, Lieberman A, Taylor RB, Waters CH. Etiology and pathogenesis. *Continuum.* 1995; 1(4):6-25.

4. Goetz CG, Jankovic J, Koller WC, Lieberman A, Taylor RB, Waters CH. Preclinical disease, differential diagnosis. *Continuum.* 1995;1(4):26-61.

2 Epidemiology

As a rule, Parkinson's disease (PD) begins between the ages of 40 and 70 years, with peak age of onset in the sixth decade. It is infrequent before 30 years of age (only 4 of 380 cases in one series[1]). Onset at younger than 20 years is known as juvenile parkinsonism, which has a different pattern of nigral degeneration and is often hereditary or caused by Huntington's or Wilson's disease.[2] PD is more common in men, with a male-to-female ratio of 3:2.

Parkinson's disease makes up approximately 80% of cases of parkinsonism. In North America there are approximately 1 million patients; about 1% of the population over the age of 65 years is afflicted.[1] The prevalence of PD is approximately 160/100,000, and the incidence is about 20/100,000.[2] But both prevalence and incidence increase with age: at age 70 years, they reach approximately 55/100,000 and 120/100,000/year, respectively.[2]

The incidence in all countries where vital statistics are kept is the same. Considering this frequency, coincidence in a family on the basis of chance occurrence might be as high as 5%.

REFERENCES

1. Adams RD, Victor M, Ropper AH. *Principles of Neurology.* 6th ed. New York, NY: McGraw-Hill; 1997:1067-1078.

2. Fahn S. Parkinsonism. In: Rowland LP, ed. *Merritt's Textbook of Neurology.* 9th ed. Baltimore, Md: Williams & Wilkins; 1995:713-730.

3 Natural History

The pathological changes of Parkinson's disease (PD) may appear as long as three decades before the appearance of clinical signs. Onset is so gradual and insidious, however, that patients rarely can pinpoint the first symptom(s). Early symptoms may be so mild that a clinical diagnosis is not possible.

According to some patients, symptoms appeared only during periods of stress, then subsided only to reappear several years later.[1] Others describe a history of disability consistent with parkinsonism that was present many years before a definite diagnosis was made. Patients' families often recall subtle motor and mental changes that antedate the diagnosis by years.

A large body of evidence indicates the progression of PD may be rapid in the preclinical stage as well as during the first years of the disease, with subsequent slowing of the process.[2] According to the Deprenyl and Tocopherol Antioxidative Therapy of Parkinsonism (DATATOP) Unified Parkinson's Disease Rating Scale study, motor examination scores declined at a rate of 8% to 9% per year in untreated patients.[3]

Correlation of the progressive disability with the biological and pathological changes in PD and the compensating mechanisms is illustrated in Figure 3.1.[4]

Before the introduction of levodopa, PD caused severe disability or death in 25% of patients within 5 years of onset, in 65% during the next 5 years, and in 89% of those surviving for 15 years.[5] The mortality rate was 3 times that of the general population matched for age, sex, and racial origin.

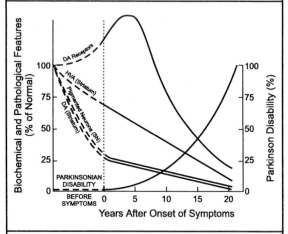

FIGURE 3.1 — THE PROGRESSIVE CHANGES IN PARKINSON'S DISEASE

In this profile of clinical, biochemical, and pathological changes in Parkinson's disease, the brain's compensating mechanisms are seen to be increases in the synthesis of dopamine receptors and turnover of surviving neurons (SN) reflected by an increase in the homovanillic acid (HVA)/dopamine (DA) ratio.

Adapted from: Jankovic J, Marsden CD. In: Jankovic J, Tolosa E, eds. *Parkinson's Disease and Movement Disorders.* 1988:95-119.

Once established, PD can follow several distinct clinical patterns. For example, two symptom-based subgroups have been noted: one dominated by postural instability and gait difficulty, a second by tremor.[6] Distinguishing features of the tremor group include:

- A family history of tremor
- Earlier age of onset
- Less functional impairment
- Preservation of mental status.

A later study questioned the more benign nature of "tremor-dominant" disease; however, in a follow-up study of 125 *de novo* PD patients (98 reassessed in 5 years),[7] a positive association was indeed found between *severity* of tremor and older age, dementia, and rapid progression of disability. But the definition of "tremor dominant" is unclear and varies in different studies, including its presence as initial symptom, chief complaint, or as only cause of disability, with no or minor rigidity or akinesia. The later findings confirm other reports that tremor is often less marked in the younger-onset patients, who often follow a benign course.

Tremor is not always present at the onset of PD, however. It occurs more commonly in patients with early-onset (40 years of age and younger) disease, whereas postural instability and gait difficulty are more dominant in patients with late-onset (70 years of age and older).

The presence or absence of dementia underlies another possible classification.[7] The percentage of patients in whom the symptom develops is controversial, ranging from 10% to 41% in a number of studies.

A third classification is based on the tempo of the disease: a benign form, found in 15% of patients, and malignant disease, with marked deterioration after a year of therapy. Finally, younger patients seem to experience a slower rate of progression but are much more troubled with motor fluctuations than their older counterparts.

Without treatment, the end stage of the illness is a rigid, akinetic state in which patients are incapable of caring for themselves. Death is usually due to complications of immobility, such as pulmonary embolism or aspiration pneumonia.

REFERENCES

1. Goetz CG, Jankovic J, Koller WC, Lieberman A, Taylor RB, Waters CH. Preclinical disease, differential diagnosis. *Continuum*. 1995;1(4):26-61.

2. Poewe WH, Wenning GK. The natural history of Parkinson's disease. *Neurology*. 1996;47(6 suppl 3):S146-S152.

3. The Parkinson Study Group. Effect of deprenyl on the progression of disability in early Parkinson's disease. *N Engl J Med*. 1989;321:1364-1371.

4. Jankovic J, Marsden CD. Therapeutic strategies in Parkinson's disease. In: Jankovic J, Tolosa E, eds. *Parkinson's Disease and Movement Disorders*. Baltimore, Md: Urban & Schwarzenberg; 1988:95-119.

5. Fahn S, Parkinsonism. In: Rowland LP, ed. *Merritt's Textbook of Neurology*. 9th ed. Baltimore, Md: Williams & Wilkins; 1995:713-730.

6. Jankovic J, McDermott M, Carter J, et al. Variable expression of Parkinson's disease: a base-line analysis of the DATATOP cohort. The Parkinson Study Group. *Neurology*. 1990;40:1529-1534.

7. Hely MA, Morris JG, Reid WG, et al. Age at onset: the major determinant of outcome in Parkinson's disease. *Acta Neurol Scand*. 1995;92:455-463.

4 Etiology

The cause of Parkinson's disease (PD), a subject rich in theories, probably is multifactorial, with contributions of variable significance from hereditary predisposition, environmental toxins, and aging. The probable contribution of endogenously generated toxic molecules is discussed in Chapter 5, *Pathogenesis.*

Aging

The fact that PD is one of the most common causes of disability among the elderly engendered two theories:

- One, that the disease is an accelerated form of aging;
- Two, that some acute exogenous or endogenous insult to the substantia nigra, followed by slow age-related nigral cell attrition leads to the onset and progression of symptoms with increasing frequency after the sixth decade.

A characteristic histologic sign of PD, the presence of Lewy bodies in the substantia nigra, appears occasionally in aging nonparkinsonian individuals, perhaps as a herald of the disease had they lived long enough.[1] Moreover, nigral cells have been shown to diminish normally with age, from about 425,000 to 200,000 by age 80 years. In PD, however, the overall number of pigmented neurons in the substantia nigra has been found to be reduced to about 31% of that in age-matched controls.

Moreover, the pathological process of PD occurs predominantly in the relatively lightly pigmented neurons of the ventrointermediate and ventrolateral regions of the substantia nigra pars compacta, whereas age-related attrition is more often seen in the dorsal tier and pars lateralis, where neuronal melanin content is somewhat greater (Figure 4.1).[2]

Thus, the speed of regional neuronal loss in aging is far less than that seen in PD (Figure 4.2) and occurs in an area opposite from that involved in PD.

Genetics

The 1990s has seen remarkable progress in the search for a genetic contribution to the pathogenesis of PD. Among the decade's findings:

- At least one first-degree relative of 20% to 25% of patients with PD has the disease or apparent essential tremor, suggesting possible genetic etiology, as well as a possible genetic association of familial essential tremor with PD.[3]
- Twin studies involving elderly male monozygotic and dizygotic twins found concordance for PD to be inconsistent with a strongly genetic etiology; however, higher concordance in younger-onset disease among monozygotic pairs suggested a substantial genetic determinant.[4]
- Reports of large families with autopsy-proven, dominantly inherited PD describe a clinical condition similar to the sporadic disease, but with earlier age of onset, more rapid progression, and a higher incidence of dementia.[5]

In 1996, an international team of investigators reported that a Parkinson disease susceptibility gene in a large Italian family afflicted by a form of the disease that develops at an early age is located on the long arm of human chromosome four. Then, in 1997, the same group identified a specific molecular alter-

4

FIGURE 4.1 — SUBREGIONAL DIVISIONS OF THE PARS COMPACTA OF THE SUBSTANTIA NIGRA

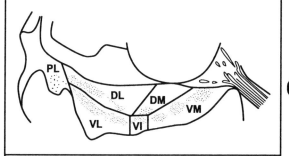

Abbreviations: PL, pars lateralis; VL, lateral ventral; DL, lateral dorsal; VI, intermediate ventral; DM, medial dorsal; VM, medial ventral.

In this schematic of the pars compacta's subregions, the distribution of pigmented nigral neurons is indicated roughly by dots of varying size and intensity. At least 60% of these neurons are lost in Parkinson's disease, particularly from the ventrolateral and ventrointermediate pars compacta. Other neurodegenerative diseases characterized by nigral lesions may also show marked neuronal loss in the ventrolateral nigra but with greater involvement of the dorsal and medial tiers as well as the striatum. Age-related loss occurs predominantly in the dorsal tier and pars lateralis, with relative sparing of the ventrolateral region.

Adapted from: Gibb WRG, Lees AJ. In: Marsden CD, Fahn S, eds. *Movement Disorders 3*. 1994:147-165.

ation in the α-synuclein gene, which codes for a presynaptic protein thought to be involved in neuronal plasticity.[6] (α-Synuclein, a presynaptic nerve terminal protein, was originally identified as the precursor protein for a component of Alzheimer's disease amyloid plaques).

This mutation is unlikely to account for most cases of sporadic, and even of familial PD, however.

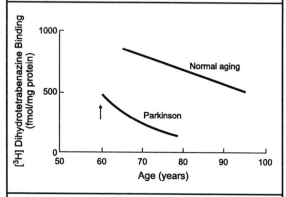

FIGURE 4.2 — COMPARISON OF AGE- AND PARKINSON'S DISEASE-RELATED NIGROSTRIATAL NEURON LOSS

The density of [³H] dihydrotetrabenazine binding sites in the caudate nucleus reflects dopaminergic innervation. In this schematic representation of age-related binding in the caudate nucleus in control subjects and in patients with onset of Parkinson's disease at age 60 years, the arrow indicates the threshold value of binding corresponding to the onset of disease.

Adapted from: Gibb WRG, Lees AJ. In: Marsden CD, Fahn S, eds. *Movement Disorders 3*. 1994:147-165.

Thus, the finding's significance is not currently clear. Nevertheless, it is currently generally acknowledged that the pathogenesis of PD requires a genetic defect, possibly with some superimposed exogenous factor.[5]

Environment

The theory that exposure to some exogenous agent may be the cause of PD was the result of the accidental intoxication of drug users by methylphenyltetrahydropyridine (MPTP), a contaminant in illicit street drugs. Patients presented with a sudden onset of all the symptoms of PD, although with less tremor and more cognitive and emotional disability, drooling, and gait and balance difficulty. Furthermore, the pathologic change characteristic of PD, the Lewy body, is not seen in experimental parkinsonism induced in primates by MPTP. Although clinical progression of MPTP-induced parkinsonism is rare, delayed-onset movement disorders have been reported in patients after transient exposure.[7]

Despite these clinical and pathological differences between the MPTP-induced condition and idiopathic PD, the use of MPTP in monkeys has provided an excellent animal model of the disease.

Actually, MPTP itself is nontoxic; rather, its oxidation product, 1-methyl-4-phenylpyridinium ion (MPP^+) is the culprit, found to be highly destructive to neurons containing melanin pigment, such as those in the substantia nigra. MPTP is oxidized to MPP^+ by monoamine oxidase type B (MAO-B), one of the isoenzymes that catabolizes dopamine. Both the oxidation and, in turn, the toxic effects of MPTP can be blocked in animals before exposure to MPTP by the administration of deprenyl (Selegiline), an MAO-B inhibitor.

Other environmental toxins that cause parkinsonism, but which affect the globus pallidus rather than the substantia nigra include:

- Carbon monoxide
- Manganese
- Carbon disulfide
- Cyanide.

A disorder with prominent substantia nigra involvement, the Parkinson disease-dementia-amyotrophic lateral sclerosis (PD-D-ALS) complex of Guam, which affects the Chamorros population of the Pacific islands Guam and Rota, has been attributed to ingestion of cycad flour.[8,9] The causative toxin has been attributed to the nonprotein amino acid β-N-methylamino-L-alanine (L-BMAA) from *Cycas circinalis* seeds. Later studies suggested the dose of BMAA ingested by the affected population would probably be insufficient to cause neurotoxicity.[10] One subsequent study has identified four other nonprotein amino acids in *Cycas circinalis* seeds, however.[11] And another, epidemiologic study associates cycasin, a mutagenic nitroso agent implicated in both the PD-D-ALS complex and diabetes mellitus in the western Pacific area.[12] The investigators conclude that further epidemiologic studies are needed to clarify the role of N-nitrosoureas in diabetes mellitus and neurodegenerative diseases in populations with different genetic backgrounds. In any case, it remains likely that the PD-D-ALS complex was caused by a toxicant.

Although a number of epidemiologic studies have found or purported to find relationships between PD and environmental exposure to a plethora of toxins, none has yet been established. Some have shown an inverse relationship between PD and smoking, suggesting tobacco may have a protective effect via an as-yet-unidentified mechanism.[13]

REFERENCES

1. Adams RD, Victor M, Ropper AH, eds. *Principles of Neurology.* 6th ed. New York, NY: McGraw-Hill; 1997:1067-1078.

2. Gibb WRG, Lees AJ. Pathological clues to the cause of Parkinson's disease. In: Marsden CD, Fahn S, eds. *Movement Disorders 3.* Oxford, UK: Butterworth-Heinemann; 1994:147-165.

3. Lazzarini AM, Myers RH, Zimmerman TR Jr, et al. A clinical genetic study of Parkinson's disease: evidence for dominant transmission. *Neurology.* 1994;44(pt 1):499-506.

4. Tanner CM, Ottman R, Ellenberg JH, et al. Parkinson's disease (PD) concordance in elderly male monozygotic (MZ) and dizygotic (DZ) twins. *Neurology*. 1997;47:A333. Abstract.

5. Golbe LI, Sage JI. Medical treatment of Parkinson's disease. In: Kurlan R, ed. *Treatment of Movement Disorders.* Philadelphia, Pa: JB Lippincott Co; 1995:1-56.

6. Polymeropoulos MH, Lavedan C, Leroy E, et al. Mutation in the α-synuclein gene identified in families with Parkinson's disease. *Science*. 1997;276:2045-2047.

7. Jankovic J. Current understanding of etiology and pathogenesis of Parkinson's disease. Syllabus, Course 127. American Academy of Neurology Annual Meeting; 1995; Seattle, Wash.

8. Spencer PS, Nunn PB, Hugon J, et al. Guam amyotrophic lateral sclerosis-parkinsonism-dementia linked to a plant excitant neurotoxin. *Science*. 1987;237:517-522.

9. Kisby GE, Ellison M, Spencer PS. Content of the neurotoxins cycasin (methylazoxymethanol beta-D-glucoside) and BMAA (beta-N-methylamino-L-alanine) in cycad flour prepared by Guam Chamorros. *Neurology*. 1992;42:1336-1340.

10. Ho SC, Woo J, Lee CM. Epidemiologic study of Parkinson's disease in Hong Kong. *Neurology*. 1989;39:1314-1318.

11. Oh CH, Brownson DM, Mabry TJ. Screening for non-protein amino acids in seeds of the Guam cycad, Cycas circinalis, by an improved GC-MS method. *Planta Med*. 1995;61:66-70.

12. Eizirik DL, Spencer P, Kisby GE. Potential role of environmental genotoxic agents in diabetes mellitus and neurodegenerative diseases. *Biochem Pharmacol*. 1996;51:1585-1591.

13. Morens DM, Grandinetti A, Waslien CI, Park CB, Ross GW, White LR. Case-control study of idiopathic Parkinson's disease and dietary vitamin E intake. *Neurology*. 1996;46:1270-1274.

4

5 Pathogenesis

The Basal Ganglia

The site of pathology responsible for the parkinsonian disorders is a group of gray matter structures within the cerebrum and ventral midbrain, the basal ganglia, generally referred to as the extrapyramidal system (Figure 5.1).[1] The basal ganglia include the:

- Striatum (caudate nucleus and putamen)
- Globus pallidus interna and externa
- Subthalamic nucleus
- Substantia nigra pars reticulata and pars compacta
- Intralaminar nuclei of the thalamus.

The *striatum* is composed of two parts, the caudate nucleus and putamen, which develop from the same telencephalic structure.[2] Fused together anteriorly, they serve as the input component of the basal ganglia.

The *globus pallidus* has two segments, the internal and external, the major output nucleus of the basal ganglia. Together the putamen and globus pallidus form a lens-shaped structure sometimes call the lenticular nucleus.

Because the *subthalamic nucleus* and the *substantia nigra* are closely linked to the striatum and globus pallidus, both anatomically and functionally, they are also considered to be basal ganglia. The subthalamic nucleus lies in the diencephalon, however, and the substantia nigra, in the mesencephalon.

The *substantia nigra* has two zones: a pale ventral area, the pars reticulata, which bears a cytologic resemblance to the globus pallidus; and a darkly pig-

31

FIGURE 5.1 — THE BASAL GANGLIA

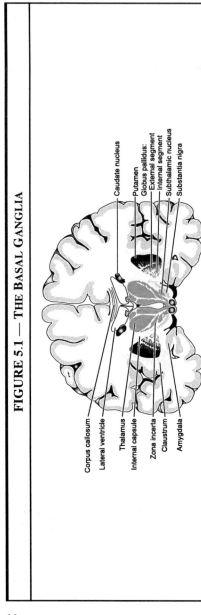

Corpus callosum
Lateral ventricle
Thalamus
Internal capsule
Zona incerta
Claustrum
Amygdala

Caudate nucleus
Putamen
Globus pallidus:
External segment
Internal segment
Subthalamic nucleus
Substantia nigra

Seen here in relation to their surrounding structures, the basal ganglia include the caudate nucleus and putamen (striatum), the globus pallidus (external and internal segments), the subthalamic nucleus, and the substantia nigra (pars compacta and pars reticulata), and the intralaminar nuclei of the thalamus.

Adapted from: Kandel ER, Schwartz JH, eds. *Principles of Neural Science.* 1985:524-531.

mented dorsal area, the pars compacta, with nerve cell bodies that contain neuromelanin, a polymer of dopamine or its metabolites (Figure 5.2).[3] The neurons of the pars compacta use dopamine as a transmitter but the function of the pigment is uncertain.

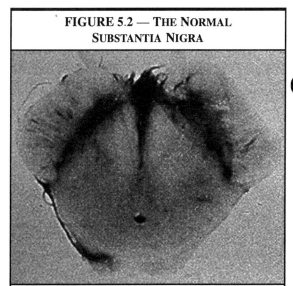

FIGURE 5.2 — THE NORMAL SUBSTANTIA NIGRA

The normal substantia nigra with its melanin-pigmented pars compacta.

Intrathalamic nuclei provide the entrance and exit pathways from the cerebral cortex to the basal ganglia and back.

The basal ganglia have separate input and output components, as well as a series of internuclear connections, mediated by specific neurotransmitters (Figure 5.3):[3] Major sources of afferent pathways arising from extrinsic neuronal groups include:

- Neocortex to the striatum, mediated by the neurotransmitter glutamate (other, as yet unidentified neurotransmitters may also be involved)

FIGURE 5.3 — MAJOR ANATOMIC PATHWAYS TO AND WITHIN THE BASAL GANGLIA

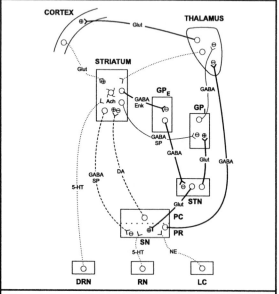

Abbreviations: GPe, globus pallidus externa; GPi, globus pallidus interna; STN, subthalamic nucleus; SNc, substantia nigra pars compacta; SNr, substantia nigra pars reticulata; DRN, dorsal raphé nucleus; RN, raphé nucleus; LC, locus ceruleus; Glut, glutamate; Ach, acetylcholine; Enk, enkephalin; GABA, gamma-aminobutyric acid; SP, substance P; 5-HT, serotonin; NE, norepinephrine.

This is a simplified version of the major connections to, among, and from the basal ganglia, including the afferent pathways from extrinsic neuronal groups (dotted lines), the striatum-SNr reciprocal pathways (broken lines), the direct pathway (heavy solid lines), the indirect pathways (solid lines), and the known excitatory (+) and inhibitory (–) transmitters.

Adapted from: Wooten GF. In: Watts RL, Koller WC, eds. *Movement Disorders: Neurologic Principles and Practice.* 1997:153-160; and, Starr MS. *Synapse.* 1995;19:264-293.

- Thalamic nonspecific nuclei to the striatum, using glutamate[4]
- Locus ceruleus to the substantia nigra, via norepinephrine
- Dorsal raphé nucleus and raphé nucleus to striatum and substantia nigra, respectively, using serotonin.

The major efferent pathways from the basal ganglia to the extrinsic neuronal groups include:

- Substantia nigra pars reticulata (SNr) and globus pallidus interna (GPi) to thalamic nuclei using gamma-aminobutyric acid (GABA)
- Thalamic nuclei to cortex, using glutamate.[4]

The nuclear groups of the basal ganglia are closely interconnected. The putamen and substantia nigra have prominent reciprocal connections mediated by specific inhibitory or excitatory neurotransmitters:[3,4]

- From striatum to SNr and GPi, mediated by the inhibitory neurotransmitter GABA and substance P (SP)
- From substantia nigra pars compacta (SNc) to striatum, mediated by dopamine (DA).

The other connections are made by two functional dopaminergic systems that are in relative balance. An indirect pathway, through which DA normally inhibits transmission, projects:[3,4]

- From striatum to globus pallidus externa (GPe), mediated by GABA and enkephalin
- From GPe to subthalamic nucleus (STN), using GABA
- From STN to SNr and GPi, using glutamate
- From SNr and GPi to ventrolateral nucleus of the thalamus, using GABA
- From thalamus to cortex, using glutamate.[4]

A direct pathway, with transmission facilitated by DA, projects from:

- Striatum to GPi, mediated by GABA and SP
- GPi to ventralis lateralis (VL) of thalamus
- Thalamus to cortex.

The striatum is driven by excitatory input from all major sensory and motor regions of the cerebral cortex, as well as the thalamic nuclei, via the excitatory thalamostriatal connection.[4] Both of these excitatory pathways use glutamate as their transmitter, with its principal targets being the inotropic AMPA (α-amino-3-hydroxy-5-methylisoxazole-4-propionic acid)- and NMDA (*N*-methyl-D-aspartate)-type glutamate receptors.

Direct striatal output via GABAergic, hence inhibitory, striatonigral and striatopallidal neurons, although normally electrically quiescent, can be driven by acetylcholine and glutamate. If glutamate or acetylcholine stimulates the direct striatal output pathway, they reduce inhibitory tone in nigrothalamic fibers, increase excitation in the feedback loop to the premotor cortex, and thereby permit movement (Figure 5.4).

On the other hand, when these same transmitters act on the indirect pathway, they bring about a sequence of events that ultimately sends exactly the opposite signals back to the cortex, thus prohibiting movement. Therefore, the net balance between glutamate's physiologic stimulant activity on the excitatory and inhibitory executive pathways of the striatum determines whether the basal ganglia issue instructions for motor acts to proceed or not.

Dopamine released from nigrostriatal neurons is envisaged as providing the fulcrum capable of shifting the glutamate balance towards hyper- or hypoactivity.

FIGURE 5.4 — NEUROTRANSMITTER BALANCE IN NORMAL AND DOPAMINE-DEPLETED BRAIN

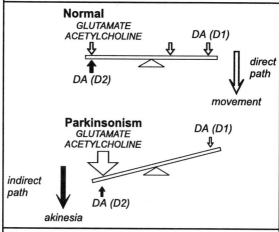

Normally, glutamate and acetylcholine activate both the direct striatal output pathway (aided by dopamine at D_1 receptors) and the indirect pathway (opposed by dopamine at D_2 receptors) output pathways, permitting movement. (Top) Loss of dopamine in the striatum upsets the finely tuned balance and, in turn, normal movement by reducing both D_1-mediated stimulation of the direct pathway and D_2-mediated inhibition of the indirect pathway. Increased presynaptic release of glutamate and acetylcholine in the striatum results in heightened impulse traffic in the GABAergic striatopallidal connection to the globus pallidus externa. The resultant disinhibition of glutamatergic neurons in the subthalamic nucleus activates the inhibitory output neurons of the substantia nigra and the globus pallidus interna, thus decreasing feedback via the thalamocortical loop (see Figure 5.3).

Adapted from: Starr MS. *Synapse*. 1995;19:264-293.

Thus, the circuitry's distinct neurotransmitter anatomy permits modulation of the motor cortex's output, apparently to aid in the generation of commands concerned with controlling proximal muscle groups during movements.[1] It monitors ongoing movement in order to prepare the motor system for the next movement in a sequence. When a particular behavior is selected, the appropriate neurons can be excited, inhibited, and disinhibited to facilitate and maintain motor programs, with emphasis on suppression of unwanted movements. The basal ganglia are instrumental in unconscious "automatic" reflexes that underlie such activities as eating, adjustment of posture, and defensive reactions.

Dopamine

Synthesized in the brain's dopaminergic neurons and other neurons from the amino acid L-tyrosine via the intermediate compound, L-3,4-dihydroxyphenylalanine (L-dopa), dopamine is then concentrated in the neurons' storage vesicles. Under physiologic conditions, dopamine is released by a calcium-dependent mechanism into the synaptic cleft, where it may bind to either (Figure 5.5):[3,5]

- Postsynaptic receptors on target cells
- Autoreceptors, specific cell surface receptors on the same neuron.

Dopamine is inactivated primarily by the reuptake process, after which it may be sequestered again in storage vesicles for release. It is also inactivated enzymatically by the action of both monoamine oxidase type B (MAO-B), an enzyme associated with mitochondria and present in two forms, A and B, and by catechol-O-methyltransferase (COMT), an enzyme localized primarily in the brain's glial cells. The principle metabolite of dopamine is homovanillic acid (HVA).

Physiologically, the striatonigral and striatal-GPe pathways appear to be excited by the action of dopamine, whereas the striatal-GPi pathway is inhibited by

FIGURE 5.5 — THE DOPAMINERGIC NEURON

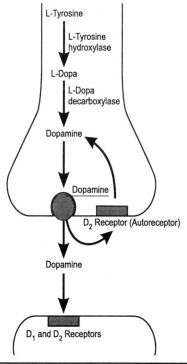

Synthesis of dopamine by dopaminergic neurons of the substantia nigra proceeds from conversion of L-tyrosine to L-dopa via L-tyrosine hydroxylase and from L-dopa to dopamine via L-dopa decarboxylase. Once synthesized, dopamine is concentrated in storage vesicles, from which, under physiological conditions, it is released into the synaptic cleft. Here, it may bind to postsynaptic D_1 and D_2 receptors in the striatum or may be inactivated by reuptake. After reuptake, dopamine may be sequestered again in storage vesicles for rerelease.

Goetz CG, et al. *Continuum*. 1995;4:7.

it. Dopamine's capacity to reverse the bradykinesia, rigidity, and tremor caused by dopamine depletion seems to require action at both receptor types.

■ Dopamine Receptors

At least six different forms of the dopamine receptor are now known, categorized under two main types D_1-like and D_2-like.[6] The D_1 type, which is generally stimulatory, is divided into two subtypes:

- D_1
- D_5.

The D_2, inhibitory, type includes:

- D_{2short}
- D_{2long}
- D_3
- D_4.

The pharmacological profile and regional distribution in brain of each subtype is different, with the exception of D_{2short} and D_{2long}, which appear to be identical in these respects.

Although it is now established that the stimulatory and inhibitory pathways act synergistically in the expression of certain behaviors, the neuroanatomical basis for the interaction is not clear. It appears, however, that striatal D_1-like receptors are expressed predominantly by striatonigral and striatopallidal neurons that are GABAergic and also express SP.[3]

In contrast, D_2-like receptors seem to be expressed primarily by substantia nigra dopaminergic neurons (autoreceptors), cholinergic interneurons in the striatum, and striatopallidal neurons projecting to the GPe, which are GABAergic and coexpress enkephalin.

■ Dopamine's Role in Parkinson's Disease

The foremost pathological characteristic of Parkinson's disease (PD) is the death of pigmented dopamine neurons in the SNc. Overt parkinsonism does not present until approximately 80% of striatal dopamine loss has occurred, however.[7] The remaining nigrostriatal neurons mount a compensatory response to severe losses by increasing the rate of dopamine synthesis and release.

Another compensatory mechanism is a reduction in the rate of dopamine inactivation. As the number of dopamine nerve terminals in the striatum decreases, so does the density of dopamine uptake sites, which comprise the primary mechanism for regulating the synaptic concentration of dopamine.[3] Thus, dopamine in the extracellular fluid can diffuse further and persist for a longer period than normal, providing the potential for it to interact with more distant postsynaptic dopamine receptors than normally.

Eventual decompensation results in an imbalance in the equilibrium between the direct and indirect striatal output pathways, however (Figure 5.5).[4] In the absence of dopamine, the driving of striatopallidal GABAergic neurons by glutamate and acetylcholine goes unchecked. The loss of D_2 inhibitory control, both pre- and postsynaptically in the striatum leads to a pronounced increase in basal ganglia inhibitory output from the indirect pathway, giving rise to the classical symptoms of rigidity and akinesia.

The Parkinson Lesion

The primary lesion of PD is degeneration of the neuromelanin-containing neurons in the brain stem, particularly those in the pars compacta of the substantia nigra, which becomes visibly pale to the naked eye (Figure 5.6). Microscopically, the pigmented nuclei show a marked depletion of cells and replacement gliosis.[5]

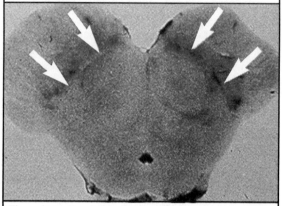
The surviving neurons are likely to contain eosinophilic cytoplasmic inclusions with peripheral halos known as Lewy bodies, the pathologic hallmark of PD[8] (Figure 5.7). By electron microscopy, the predominant structural component of the Lewy body is seen to be filamentous material arranged in circular and linear profiles, sometimes radiating from an electron-dense core. A weakly staining second inclusion called a pale body is also found frequently but not invariably. It consists of a very sparse accumulation of neurofilament interspersed with vacuoles and granular bodies. The cause of this excessive accumulation of filamentous material within surviving neurons is unknown.

Although Lewy bodies are present in PD, they are also found in a few other rare neurodegenerative diseases. The most recently recognized of these, diffuse Lewy body disease (DLBD), is differentiated from PD by widespread cortical and subcortical Lewy body for-

FIGURE 5.7 — THE LEWY BODY

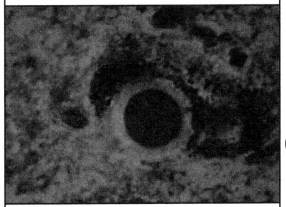

Lewy bodies are rounded, eosinophilic, intracytoplasmic neuronal inclusions classically associated with Parkinson's disease. They are found in selected brainstem nuclei (substantia nigra, locus ceruleus, dorsal vagal nucleus), the nucleus basalis of Meynert, hypothalamus, and sympathetic ganglia.

mation and the invariable development of dementia. Patients usually present with a neurobehavioral syndrome, which may include hallucinations, delusions, and psychosis, and all eventually become demented. The second most common cause of dementia after Alzheimer's disease, DLBD has been suggested as one extreme of the spectrum of PD, with the proposed pathological classification:[8]

- Type A, diffuse disease with numerous Lewy bodies in brain stem and cortex
- Type B, the transitional form, with many brain stem and diencephalic, fewer cortical Lewy bodies
- Type C, the brain stem form, with few if any cortical Lewy bodies.

Types B and C are consistent with PD.

REFERENCES

1. Kandel ER, Schwartz JH, eds. *Principles of Neural Science.* 2nd ed. New York, NY: Elsevier; 1985:524-531.

2. Nolte J, ed. *The Human Brain: An Introduction to Its Functional Anatomy.* 2nd ed. St. Louis, Mo: The CV Mosby Company; 1988.

3. Wooten GF. Neurochemistry and neuropharmacology of Parkinson's disease. In: Watts RL, Koller WC, eds. *Movement Disorders: Neurologic Principles and Practice.* New York, NY: McGraw-Hill; 1997:153-160.

4. Starr MS. Glutamate/dopamine D_1/D_2 balance in the basal ganglia and its relevance to Parkinson's disease. *Synapse.* 1995;19:264-293.

5. Goetz CG, Jankovic J, Koller WC, Lieberman A, Taylor RB, Waters CH. Etiology and pathogenesis. *Continuum.* 1995; 1(4):6-25.

6. Elsworth JD, Roth RH. Dopamine synthesis, uptake, metabolism, and receptors: relevance to gene therapy of Parkinson's disease. *Exp Neurol.* 1997;144:4-9.

7. Jankovic J, Marsden CD. Therapeutic strategies in Parkinson's disease. In: Jankovic J, Tolosa E, eds. *Parkinson's Disease and Movement Disorders.* Baltimore, Md: Urban & Schwarzenberg; 1988:95-119.

8. Kalra S, Bergeron C, Lang AE. Lewy body disease and dementia. A review. *Arch Intern Med.* 1996;156:487-493.

6   Pathophysiology

Although the cause of the nigral neuronal destruction in Parkinson's disease (PD) remains unknown, studies of the substantia nigra after death in PD patients has identified three major changes:[1]

- Evidence of oxidative stress and depletion of reduced glutathione
- High levels of total iron with reduced ferritin buffering
- Mitochondrial complex I deficiency.

The Oxidative Stress Hypothesis

Oxidative, or oxidant stress occurs when the equilibrium between antioxidant defense mechanisms and factors that promote free radical formation is disturbed.[2] Because aerobic cells use molecular oxygen as the terminal electron acceptor in oxidative phosphorylation, they must be capable of dealing with the side effects of oxygen and its reactive derivatives. These are, in order of reduction from oxygen:

- Superoxide anion radical
- Hydrogen peroxide
- Hydroxy radicals.

Under physiologic conditions, superoxide is readily reduced to hydrogen peroxide, oxygen, and water by enzymes such as superoxide dismutase, catalase, and glutathione peroxidase or by interaction with transitional metals. Although peroxide is relatively unreactive towards organic compounds, its interaction with transitional metals (copper, iron) generates the more reactive hydroxyl radical, reported to induce apoptosis (see below) in rat cortical neurons. Hydroxyl radicals are highly toxic and can combine with or abstract moieties from practically any biological molecule, including DNA, protein, and lipid membranes.

In addition to reduction by enzymes, free radicals are opposed or destroyed by several defense mechanisms, which include:

- A number of antioxidant molecules present in the tissues, among which glutathione assumes major importance
- Scavengers such as vitamin E and ascorbate, which react directly with free radicals to prohibit their damaging effects
- Proteins such as transferrin and ferritin, which bind and maintain iron in a relatively nonreactive state
- The proto-oncogene *bel-2*, mainly localized to the mitochondrial membrane, which blocks apoptosis through reduced generation of the reactive oxygen species.

The brain appears to be particularly vulnerable to oxidative stress. Neuronal membranes contain a high proportion of radical-susceptible polyunsaturated fatty acid. Moreover, the brain's antioxidant defenses are weak, with low levels of glutathione, almost no catalase, and comparatively low concentrations of glutathione peroxidase and vitamin E. Add to this the brain's relatively high oxygen consumption and its susceptibility to physiologic disequilibrium with resultant oxidative stress, and free radical damage becomes clear.

Because the substantia nigra is rich in dopamine, which can undergo both monoamine oxidase (MAO)-mediated enzymatic oxidation and auto-oxidation to neuromelanin, hydrogen peroxide and free radicals are generated in its neurons. Normally, lipid peroxidation can be quenched by vitamin E (alpha tocopherol), or by the enzyme glutathione peroxidase, which removes hydrogen peroxide and lipid peroxides.[3] In the process, hydrogen peroxide, in conjunction with glutathione peroxidase, transforms the enzyme's cosubstrate, glutathione (GSH) to form oxidized glutathione disulfide (GSSG). Reduced glutathione is regenerated by the action of glutathione reductase.[4]

Only trace concentrations of GSH (1% of total glutathione) are normally present in the brain, but levels increase with oxidant stress. The cellular level of GSSG depends on the balance between the rate at which it is formed and that at which it reverts back to GSH under the influence of GSSG reductase. In this way, peroxide-mediated changes in glutathione could conceivably arise from levodopa therapy. Furthermore, quinones derived from levodopa make irreversible addition products with GSH, which permanently remove GSH from further participation in cellular defense mechanisms.[3]

A controlled, comparative study of GSH and GSSG levels in the brains of patients who died of PD and those who died with progressive supranuclear palsy (PSP), Huntington's disease, and multiple system atrophy (MSA) revealed a significant (40%) decrease in GSH only in Parkinson's brain; this in spite of the fact that profound nigral cell loss was seen in the substantia nigra of Parkinson's, MSA and PSP brains.[5] No other changes in glutathione content were found elsewhere in the Parkinson brains. These findings suggest that the change in PD is not due solely to nigral cell death. Finally, the GSH/GSSG nigral ratio, which ranged from a high 226-800:1 in controls, was significantly altered in favor of GSSG in Parkinson nigral cells.

Given the dopamine-free radical connection, however, an interesting question continues to arise: Does

L-dopa therapy contribute to the glutathione changes in the Parkinson brain?[3] A contribution from levodopa therapy cannot be ruled out for the observed change in GSH/GSSG ratio.

■ Apoptosis

The mode of neuron death in degenerative diseases is now thought to be via apoptosis, a morphologically unique process of cell death distinctly different from necrosis. Necrosis is accidental death resulting from severe and sudden thermal, physical, or chemical trauma and characterized by early mitochondrial and cellular swelling, with ensuing cytoskeletal disruption and ruptured plasma membrane and organelles. The nuclear structure remains intact.

Apoptosis is a sequential process that starts with condensation of chromatin and shrinkage of cell volume.[6] The plasma membrane becomes ruffled and blebbed. Nucleus and cytoplasm are partitioned into membrane-bound apoptotic bodies that are shed from the dying cells. In the last stages, most cells display a characteristic degradation of nuclear DNA into multimers of 180 bp (DNA laddering). Throughout the process, the mitochondria remain morphologically normal. The dying cell is subsequently phagocytosed by neighboring cells.

Neurons die by apoptosis during development of the brain. Apoptosis can be induced by removal of trophic factors from primary cultures of neurons.[2] The apoptotic pathway is regulated by the levels of certain apoptosis-related genes. For example, the level of *bel-2* can determine the sensitivity of neurons to glutamate excitotoxicity and trophic factor deprivation. The pro-aptotic gene p53 can have the opposite effect.

The involvement of apoptosis in neurodegenerative diseases was confirmed by exposure of cultured neurons to a range of conditions characteristic of those disorders, all of which induce cell death by apoptosis:

- Glutathione depletion
- Chronic inhibition of superoxide dismutase
- β-Amyloid fragments
- Dopamine
- Ischemia.

Although apoptosis is commonly equated with programmed cell death in vertebrate systems, a genetic program has been established unequivocally in only a small worm (Caenorhabditis elegans).[6]

Iron

Defective iron uptake and storage is among the most prominent biochemical features of neurodegeneration.[7] Because free iron can facilitate decompensation of lipid peroxides and formation of hydroxyl radicals, close cellular regulation allows only a small percentage of the overall iron store to be available in free ionic form. If not used by enzymes as a cofactor, it is largely bound to the storage and transport proteins, ferritin and transferrin, respectively, or to low molecular weight chelators such as adenosine triphosphate (ATP), adenosine 5'-diphosphate (ADP), and citrate. Transferrins are the main iron-binding proteins in body fluids.

Immunohistochemical data show little or no ferritin in neurons throughout the brain. Thus, the metal ions required for metabolic processes must be predominantly in free form. However, the neuromelanin in dopaminergic nigrostriatal neurons has two populations of binding sites for ferric iron, thus can serve as a buffer for free iron.

The involvement of iron in the development and progression of neurodegenerative disease is strongly suggested by the finding of a marked increase of iron in Parkinson brains as well as those affected by Huntington's disease, supranuclear palsy, multisystem atrophy, and Alzheimer's disease. The reason for this toxic buildup has yet to be established. The secondary role of iron accumulation cannot be ruled out; however, strong evidence of a direct contribution to the progression of neurodegeneration includes:

- Parkinson-like behavior responses as well as the typical ipsilateral decrease in dopamine concentration has been induced by unilateral injection of iron into the substantia nigra of rats.
- Increased brain iron can lead to oxidative stress (interaction with peroxide generates hydroxyl radical), thus causing free radical-induced neurodegeneration.
- In the presence of excess free iron, the antioxidant neuromelanin releases free iron to participate with peroxide in the formation of free radicals.

Peripheral metabolism of iron is apparently unrelated to the risk of developing PD. In 68 patients and controls, a single intramuscular injection of desferrioxamine, 1 mg/kg, resulted in no significant differences in serum levels of iron transferrin and ferritin or in 24-hour urine iron excretion.

Mitochondrial Injury

The first clue to the possibility of mitochondrial dysfunction in PD came with an understanding of MPTP's (methylphenyltetrahydropyridine) mechanism of action.[8] After conversion by monoamine oxidase type B (MAO-B), the neurotoxin's product, methyl phenylpyridinium ion (MPP+), is actively taken up into dopaminergic neurons and concentrated in mitochondria. Here, it specifically inhibits complex I ($NADH\ CoQ_1$) reductase, the first enzyme of the respiratory chain. The resulting decrease in ATP synthesis is thought to account for the death of the dopamine-containing neurons.

Analysis of respiratory chain activity in the Parkinson brain has shown a 37% decrease in complex I activity, with normal activity in complexes II to IV. This selective deficiency of complex I activity seems to be confined to the substantia nigra, particularly the pars compacta.[9]

These observations led to studies of mitochondrial function in non-neural tissues, such as platelets, which have been seen as a mirror of biochemical processes in the brain. In most studies, platelet complex I activity was found to be significantly lower in Parkinson disease patients than in controls.[8,10]

Glutathione has been suggested as a link between the main pathogenetic hypotheses of neurodegeneration in PD: oxidative stress and mitochondrial injury.[11] Although most glutathione is localized in the cytosolic fraction, approximately 10% is compartmentalized within mitochondria, which also contain the complete enzymatic system, including GSH, for detoxication of hydroperoxides. Glutathione is also likely to be involved in maintaining intramitochondrial protein thiols in a reduced state. Thiols are essential to a number of the organelles' functions, including selective membrane permeability and calcium homeostasis. Thus excessive production of peroxide within mitochondria could lead to depletion of GSH, oxidation of protein thiols, and impairment of mitochondrial function.

Since mitochondrial GSH originates from the cytosol, any significant decrease in cellular levels of glutathione is likely to affect mitochondrial function.[11] If loss of GSH can cause mitochondrial damage, it is also conceivable that impairment of mitochondrial function can lead to a decrease in cytosolic GSH. Glutathione synthesis requires ATP and thus a deficiency of energy supplied by mitochondria is likely to affect the cellular turnover of glutathione.

Given the association of MPP^+ with parkinsonism, the mechanism by which it causes a decrease in GSH levels may be relevant in interpreting the loss of glutathione seen in the parkinsonian brain and may point to deficient mitochondrial activity as a possible initial event. Consequent impairment of glutathione turnover may then contribute to make dopaminergic neurons of the substantia nigra particularly susceptible to oxidative damage. Regardless of the initial insult, a cascade of events involving both oxygen radicals and mitochondrial metabolism is likely to contribute to cell injury.

Excitatory Amino Acids and Oxidative Stress

At about the time the excitatory amino acids (EAAs) glutamate, aspartate, and related compounds were identified as the predominant neurotransmitters of the central nervous system (CNS), the EAAs neurotoxic properties were also being explored.[12] Intracerebral injection of the EAAs into mice destroyed neurons in the area of injection, with neurotoxicity mediated through inotropic EAA neurotransmitter receptors.

These receptors have been classified according to the glutamate analogues that are most specific in exciting defined physiologic responses:
- AMPA (α-amino-3-hydroxy-5-methyl-4-isoxasolproprionate)
- NMDA (N-methyl-D-aspartate)
- Kainate.

Although all three receptors can initiate neurotoxicity, there has been particularly strong interest in the NMDA/glutamate subtype, which has unusual physiologic properties:

- The postsynaptic potential produced by receptor activation has slower onset and longer duration than that of the other two.
- Its postsynaptic potential exhibits voltage dependency; at normal resting membrane potential it is difficult to activate but becomes increasingly easy to activate as the membrane becomes depolarized.

6

Although the etiology of nerve cell death in neuronal degenerative diseases, including PD, is unknown, one hypothesis holds that excitotoxic mechanisms may play a role.[13] In the normal brain, concentration of EAAs are maintained within the synaptic cleft at subtoxic levels, with rapid uptake and inactivation by both neurons and glia. However, a defect in mitochondrial function, specifically diminished activity of complex I of the electron transport chain, presumably causes a bioenergetic defect in the dopamine neurons of the substantia nigra, reducing their capacity to maintain a normal membrane potential. Thus, voltage-dependent NMDA ion channels are more easily activated, leading to slow excitotoxic neuronal death.

Evidence Against the Oxidative Stress Hypothesis

The hypothesis that damage to the neuronal cells of the substantia nigra by free radicals is responsible for the pathogenesis of PD, although generally accepted, has been questioned on several clinical and laboratory grounds.[14]

Clinical questions are based on the absence of:

- A deleterious effect of L-dopa therapy, which has not been shown to accelerate neuronal loss; side effects are all dose-dependent and reversible
- An obvious impact of the MAO inhibitor deprenyl (selegiline) on the progress of the disease[15]
- Increasing asymmetry in PD; compensatory synthesis of dopamine should cause increased dopamine turnover and, in turn increased free radical damage on the side with greatest neuronal degeneration.[14]

Laboratory-related questions involve the absence of:

- The correlation between rates of dopamine turnover and dopaminergic cell death; neuronal loss should be highest in brain areas where dopamine turnover rate is maximal but no such relationship has been found
- A correlation between melanin content and neuronal vulnerability; if melanin binds metals that catalyze production of free radicals, pigmented neurons should be the most vulnerable, but predominant neural loss has been found in the substantia nigra region with low neuronal melanin content
- A general loss of dopaminergic cells; cell loss is localized to neurons of the ventrolateral substantia nigra with sparing of those in other brain and peripheral areas
- A "free radical" explanation for other neurodegenerative disorders that share features of PD
- An effect of deprenyl on indices of free radical scavenging in PD.

Thus, despite the popularity of the free radical hypothesis and its suggestion of a therapeutic potential for neuroprotection, it poses a number of problems that must be addressed. According to one cautious critic, "it is equally likely that in some (perhaps most) diseases, the increased oxidant formation is an epiphenomenon that makes no significant contribution to the progression of the disease."[16]

REFERENCES

1. Jenner P, Schapira AH, Marsden CD. New insights into the cause of Parkinson's disease. *Neurology*. 1992;42:2241-2250.

2. Gorman AM, McGowan A, O'Neill C, Cotter T. Oxidative stress and apoptosis in neurodegeneration. *J Neurol Sci*. 1996;139(suppl):45-52.

3. Cohen G. The brain on fire. *Ann Neurol*. 1994;36:333-334. Editorial.

4. Jenner P, Dexter DT, Sian J, Schapira AH, Marsden CD. Oxidative stress as a cause of nigral cell death in Parkinson's disease and incidental Lewy body disease. The Royal Kings and Queens Parkinson's Disease Research Group. *Ann Neurol*. 1992;32(suppl):S82-S87.

5. Sian J, Dexter DT, Lees AJ, et al. Alterations in glutathione levels in Parkinson's disease and other neurodegenerative disorders affecting basal ganglia. *Ann Neurol*. 1994;36:348-355.

6. Lee WMF, Dang CV. Control of cell growth, differentiation, and death. In: Hoffman R, Benz EJ Jr, Shattil SJ, Furie B, Cohen HJ, Silberstein LE, eds. *Hematology: Basic Principles and Practice*. 2nd ed. New York, NY: Churchill Livingstone; 1995:81.

7. Gassen M, Youdim MBH. The potential role of iron chelators in the treatment of Parkinson's disease and related neurological disorders. *Pharmacol Toxicol*. 1997;80:159-166.

8. Krige D, Carroll MT, Cooper JM, Marsden CD, Schapira AH. Platelet mitochondrial function in Parkinson's disease. The Royal Kings and Queens Parkinson's Disease Research Group. *Ann Neurol*. 1992;32:782-788.

9. Schapira AH, Mann VM, Cooper JM, Krige D, Jenner PJ, Marsden CD. Mitochondrial function in Parkinson's disease. The Royal Kings and Queens Parkinson's Disease Research Group. *Ann Neurol*. 1992;32(suppl):S116-S124.

10. Shults CW, Nasirian F, Ward DM, et al. Carbidopa/levodopa and selegiline do not affect platelet mitochondrial function in early parkinsonism. *Neurology*. 1995;45:344-348.

11. Di Monte DA, Chan P, Sandy MS. Glutathione in Parkinson's disease: a link between oxidative stress and mitochondrial damage? *Ann Neurol*. 1992;32(suppl):S111-S115.

12. Albin RL, Greenamyre JT. Alternative excitotoxic hypotheses. *Neurology*. 1992;42:733-738.

13. Beal MF. Does impairment of energy metabolism result in excitotoxic neuronal death in neurodegenerative illnesses? *Ann Neurol*. 1992;31:119-130.

14. Calne DB. The free radical hypothesis in idiopathic parkinsonism: evidence against it. *Ann Neurol*. 1992;32:799-803.

15. Parkinson Study Group. Impact of deprenyl and tocopherol treatment on Parkinson's disease in DATATOP patients requiring levodopa. *Ann Neurol*. 1996;39:37-45.

16. Halliwell B. Tell me about free radicals, doctor: a review. *J R Soc Med*. 1989;82:747-752.

7 Diagnosis

The cardinal signs and symptoms of Parkinson's disease (PD), when present in their entirety, impart the well-known, unmistakable clinical picture of resting tremor, rigidity, akinesia, and impairment of postural reflexes. It evolves slowly, however, with early symptoms so mild as to escape notice by either patients or those close to them. This prediagnostic period may last for years.

Initial presentation is seldom the full-blown disease. Individual physical findings are not specific to the disease; each may herald one or more long-latency parkinsonian syndromes.[1] In many cases, therefore, PD is a diagnosis of exclusion rather than a straightforward presentation of a specific deficit profile.

The diagnostic approach has been categorized as:[2]

- Clinically possible PD, the presence of any one of the salient features:
  - Tremor (resting)
  - Rigidity
  - Bradykinesia
  - Impairment of postural reflexes
- Clinically probable PD, combination of any two cardinal features (including impaired postural reflexes); alternatively, any one of the first three if asymmetrical
- Clinically definite, any combination of three of the four features; alternatively, any two with one of first three displaying asymmetry.

When not all the signs are evident, there is no alternative but to re-examine the patient at several-month intervals until it is clear that PD is present or the signature of another degenerative process becomes evident. Early in the course of the disease, when only a slight asymmetry of stride or clumsiness in one hand is present, a number of small signs may be helpful toward a clinically possible diagnosis:[3]

- A Meyerson sign (inability to avoid blinking to tap on nose or glabella)
- Digital impedance (tendency for rapid alternating movements to block or to assume a tremor rhythm)
- Lack of arm swing
- Lack of the Babinski sign or of increased tendon reflexes in affected limbs eliminates corticospinal lesion
- Lack of grasp reflex helps to exclude a premotor cerebral disorder.

As the disease progresses a number of other signs and symptoms may become apparent (Table 7.1).

Parkinson's disease can probably be excluded early with the presence of:

- Early dementia and autonomic disorder
- Ataxia and corticospinal signs.

Clinical Diagnosis

The main difficulty in the clinical diagnosis of PD is to distinguish the disease from the parkinsonian syndromes as well as other conditions that resemble specific features of either.[3] These include:

- Essential tremor
- Binswanger's disease
- Normal pressure hydrocephalus
- Progressive supranuclear palsy
- Striatonigral degeneration
- Anergic, or hypokinetic depression
- Drug-induced parkinsonism.

TABLE 7.1 — MOTOR AND NONMOTOR SYMPTOMS OF PARKINSON'S DISEASE

Motor
- Gait and axial structures
  - Altered axial posture
  - Difficulty turning in bed
  - Slow, shuffling gait
  - Propulsion and festination
- Upper and lower extremities
  - Micrographia
  - Impaired fine movements
  - Rest tremor
  - Foot and toe dystonia
- Cranial structures
  - Masked facies
  - Soft, hesitant or dysarthric speech
  - Decreased eye blinking
  - Impaired ocular accommodation
  - Blepharospasm (forced eye closure)
  - Dysphagia (swallowing dysfunction)
  - Drooling

Nonmotor
- Psychiatric and sleep
  - ?Premorbid personality
  - Depression
  - Anxiety
  - Vivid dreams
  - Sleep fragmentation
- Sensory
  - Numbness, tingling
  - Paresthesias: sensory, thermal
  - Akathisia (sensation of restlessness)
  - Olfactory deficit (smell)
  - Impaired visual contract sensitivity
- Autonomic
  - Orthostatic hypotension
  - Impaired gastrointestinal motility
  - Urinary bladder dysfunction
  - Disordered thermoregulation
  - Diminished reflex pupillary response
  - Seborrheic dermatitis
  - Weight loss
  - Sexual dysfunction

7

- **Essential Tremor** (Figure 7.1)

This heredofamilial action tremor that usually begins in early adult life and is distinguished from that of PD by:[3]

- Its low amplitude and higher frequency
- A tendency to become manifest during volitional movement and to disappear when the limb is in repose
- Lack of associated slowness of movement, flexed postures, etc.

Some slower, alternating forms of essential tremor are difficult to distinguish from parkinsonian tremor. Comparative characteristics of the two are listed in Table 7.2.[1]

FIGURE 7.1 — ESSENTIAL TREMOR

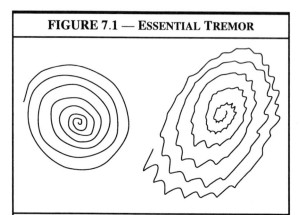

Shown here are Archimedes spirals, drawn from inside outward with at least five turns, produced by a healthy control subject (left) and a patient with essential tremor (right).

From: Bain PG, Findley LJ. *Assessing Tremor Severity.* London, UK: Smith-Gordon and Company Limited; 1993.

TABLE 7.2 — COMPARISON OF PARKINSON'S DISEASE AND ESSENTIAL TREMOR		
	Parkinson's Disease	Essential Tremor
Characteristics		
Family history	Usually negative	Positive in 50%
Alcohol	± Effect	Marked tremor reduction
Medical attention sought	Early in course	Often late in course
Age at onset	Mid-adulthood	Childhood, adulthood, or elderly
Tremor type	Resting	Postural, kinetic
Body part affected	Hands, legs	Hands, head, voice
Disease course	Progressive	Slowly progressive; static for long periods
Bradykinesia, rigidity, postural instability	May be present	Never present
Treatment		
Levodopa	Effective	No effect
Propranolol	May decrease tremor	Effective
Primidone	No effect	Effective

Adapted from: Goetz CG, et al. *Continuum.* 1995;1(4):47.

7

■ Postencephalitic Parkinsonism

Since no definite instance of encephalitis lethargica has been recorded since 1930, it is safe to say that postencephalitic parkinsonism has disappeared. Rarely, a Parkinson-like syndrome has been described associated with other forms of encephalitis, particularly that due to Japanese B virus.

■ Binswanger's Disease

A condition characterized by many infarcts and lacunes in the white matter with relative sparing of the cortex and basal ganglia, Binswanger's disease can cause a pseudobulbar palsy that presents a clinical picture simulating certain aspects of PD such as slowness and rigidity. However, unilateral and bilateral corticospinal tract signs, hyperactive facial reflexes, spasmodic crying and laughing, and other characteristic features distinguish spastic bulbar palsy from PD.

■ Normal-Pressure Hydrocephalus

Normal-pressure hydrocephalus can create a Parkinson-like condition, with gait and postural instability and, at times, bradykinesia.

■ Progressive Supranuclear Palsy

This parkinson-plus syndrome is characterized by rigidity and dystonic postures of the neck and shoulders, a staring and immobile countenance, and a tendency to topple when walking, all suggestive of Parkinson's disease. However, the diagnosis of progressive supranuclear palsy can be established in most cases by patients' inability to produce vertical saccades; paralysis of first downward, and then later, upward gaze; and eventually, paralysis of lateral gaze with retention of reflex eye movements.

Postmortem examinations have disclosed bilateral loss of neurons and gliosis in the periaqueductal gray matter, the superior colliculus, subthalamic nucleus, red nucleus, globus pallidus, dentate nucleus, pretectal and vestibular nuclei, and to some extent, the oculomotor nucleus. In some cases the neurons of the cerebral cortex have been involved but the cerebellar cortex is usually spared.

■ Striatonigral Degeneration

Also a parkinson-plus disorder (in the multiple system atrophy category), striatonigral degeneration is clinically similar to PD, with the typical rigidity, stiffness, and bradykinesia. Although postmortem examination reveals extensive loss of neurons in the pars compacta of the substantia nigra, no Lewy bodies are found in the remaining cells. Unlike the localized picture in PD, degenerative changes are also seen in the striatal putamen and caudate nuclei, findings similar to Huntington's disease. Moreover, these structures are greatly reduced in size and have lost most of their neurons. Secondary loss of striatopallidal fibers is also seen. Widespread olivopontocerebellar degeneration and argyrophilic glial inclusions have also been reported.

The clinical picture is also unlike PD, with the early appearance of severe atypical progressive parkinsonism characterized by bilateral bradykinesia and rigidity, slowness of gait, postural instability and falls, and poor or absent response to levodopa, as well as increased tendon reflexes associated or not with frank pyramidal signs.[5]

■ Multiple System Atrophy

These disorders, which represent a major subcategory of the parkinson-plus diseases, include conditions demonstrating a combination of varying degrees of parkinsonism (due to striatonigral degeneration), autonomic dysfunction (degeneration of sympathetic motor neurons), and ataxia (olivopontocerebellar degeneration).

Five features that distinguish multiple system atrophy with a pure parkinsonian presentation from PD are:[6]

- More rapid progression in multiple system atrophy
- Symmetrical onset
- Absence of tremor
- Lack of response to dopaminergic therapy (probably due to striatal damage and ensuing loss of post-synaptic receptors)
- Severe and early autonomic dysfunction.

Nearly half of the patients have orthostatic hypotension, impotence, loss of sweating, dry mouth, and miosis, shown at autopsy to be associated with loss of intermediolateral horn cells and pigmented nuclei of the brainstem (Shy-Drager syndrome).

Although these criteria are not significantly different from those for progressive supranuclear palsy, the latter can be differentiated by its clinical hallmark, early down-gaze palsy, and by axial dystonia.

The distinctive clinical profiles of PD and the four major parkinsonism-plus diseases discussed above are compared in Table 7.3.[1]

■ **Anergic Depression**

Also called hypokinetic depression, this disorder may be associated with paucity of movement, unchanging attitudes, and postural sets, and a slightly stiff and unbalanced gait. Because a high percentage of patients with PD are also depressed, initial differentiation of the two can be difficult[3] (see Chapter 9, *Complications of Parkinson's Disease and Its Therapy*).

TABLE 7.3 — COMPARISON OF PARKINSON'S AND PARKINSON-PLUS DISEASES

	Parkinson's Disease	Olivoponto-cerebellar Degeneration	Shy-Drager Syndrome	Progressive Supranuclear Palsy	Striatonigral Degeneration
Tremor	+++	+	+	+	+
Rigidity	+++	+++	+++	+++	+++
Bradykinesia	+++	+++	+++	+++	+++
Postural instability	+++	+++	+++	+++	+++
Pyramidal signs	0	0	0	+	+++
Cerebellar signs	0	+++	++	+	+
Autonomic dysfunction	++	++	+++	+	++
Dementia	++	+	+	+++	+
Axial and nuchal dystonia	0	0	0	+++	0
Supranuclear gaze palsy	0	0	0	+++	0
Response to levodopa	Good	Absent	Poor	Poor	Poor

Key: 0 = does not occur; + = rare; ++ = common; +++ = frequent.

Adapted from: Goetz CG, et al. *Continuum.* 1995;1(4):37.

■ Lewy Body Disease

Finally, differential diagnosis must include diffuse Lewy body disease, not much of a problem unless the patient is among the rare few, usually with advanced disease, who present with dementia. Although cognitive decline is a common feature of PD, it is not like the dementia seen in diffuse Lewy body and Alzheimer's disease (see Chapter 9, *Complications of Parkinson's Disease and Its Therapy*).[3]

■ Drug-Induced Parkinsonism

Many drugs can induce parkinsonism, among them (Tables 7.4, 7.5):[7]
- The neuroleptics
- The antihypertensive reserpine
- The cardiac antiarrhythmic agent amiodarone.

Although neuroleptics are used primarily as antipsychotic agents, they have a number of other, nonpsychotic uses:
- Depression
- Anxiety
- Insomnia
- Nausea and vomiting (prochlorperazine and related agents).

Metoclopromide, an atypical neuroleptic belonging to the benzamide class, is used to ameliorate gastric stasis and as an antiemetic. Various extrapyramidal reactions, including parkinsonism, have been associated with its use.

Drug-induced parkinsonism may be clinically indistinguishable from Parkinson's disease. Akinesia, rigidity, postural abnormalities, and tremor may be present. Bradykinesia is the earliest, most common and often the only manifestation, accounting for the expressionless face, loss of associated movements, slow initiation of motor activity, and disturbed speech.

TABLE 7.4 — NEUROLEPTICS AND RELATED AGENTS

Trade Name	Generic Name
Phenothiazines	
Compazine	Prochlorperazine
Etrafon, Triavil	Perphenazine and amitriptyline
Levoprome	Methotrimeprazine
Mellaril	Thioridazine
Phenergan	Promethazine
Prolixin	Fluphenazine
Norzine, Torecan	Thiethylperazine
Serentil	Mesoridazine
Sparine	Promazine
Stelazine	Trifluoperazine
Thorazine	Chlorpromazine
Trilafon	Perphenazine
Butyrophenones	
Haldol	Haloperidol
Fentanyl	Droperidol
Thioxanthenes	
Navane	Thiothixene
Taractan	Chlorprothixene
Benzamide	
Reglan	Metoclopramide
Dihydroindolone	
Moban	Molindone
Dibenzoxazepine	
Loxitane	Loxapine
Dibenzodiazepine	
Clozaril	Clozapine
Benzisoxazole	
Risperdal	Risperidone
Thienobenzodiazepine	
Olanzapine	Zyprexa

Adapted from: Hubble JP. In: Watts RL, Koller WC, eds. *Movement Disorders: Neurologic Principles and Practice.* 1997.

TABLE 7.5 — MISCELLANEOUS DRUGS ASSOCIATED WITH PARKINSONISM

- Reserpine
  - Tetrabenazine
- α-Methyldopa
- Calcium-channel blockers
  - Cinnarizine
  - Flunarizine
- Amiodarone
- Bethanechol
- Pyridostigmine
- Lithium
- Diazepam
- Fluoxetine
- Phenelzine
- Procaine
- Meperidine
- Amphotericin B
- Cephaloridine
- 5-Fluorouracil
- Vincristine-Adriamycin

Adapted from: Hubble JP. In: Watts RL, Koller WC, eds. *Movement Disorders: Neurologic Principles and Practice*. 1997.

Rigidity of the extremities, neck, or trunk, usually without a "cogwheel" phenomenon, may occur after the onset of bradykinesia. Although the characteristic parkinsonian "pill-rolling" tremor at rest may be present, postural tremor resembling essential tremor may also be seen.

Some differentiating characteristics may be present, however (Table 7.6).

Laboratory Findings

Although a number of approaches to preclinical detection of PD have been investigated, a practical, inexpensive, sensitive, specific screen test has yet to be made available. Furthermore, in the absence of a

TABLE 7.6 — DIFFERENTIAL DIAGNOSIS OF DRUG-INDUCED PARKINSONISM AND PARKINSON'S DISEASE

	Drug-Induced Parkinsonism	Parkinson's Disease
Symptom onset	Bilateral and symmetric	Unilateral or asymmetric
Course	Acute or subacute	Insidious, chronic
Tremor type	Bilateral symmetric postural or rest tremor	Unilateral or asymmetric rest tremor
Anticholinergic drug response	May be pronounced	Usually mild to moderate
Withdrawal of suspected offending drug	Remittance within weeks to months	Symptoms and signs slowly progress

Adapted from: Hubble JP. In: Watts RL, Koller WC, eds. *Movement Disorders: Neurologic Principles and Practice.* 1997.

7

disease-specific biologic marker, a definitive diagnosis of PD can be made only at autopsy. (Two separate pathological studies concluded that only 76% of clinically diagnosed Parkinson's patients actually met the pathologic criteria; 24% had other causes of parkinsonism.[8])

Of the number of possible peripheral markers of PD that have been investigated, a few show some promise, among them:

- Decrease of D_3 dopamine receptor mRNA expression as well as reduction in D_3 receptor binding sites in lymphocytes of Parkinson disease patients[9]
- Morphologic abnormalities in platelets in both treated and untreated disease[10]
- Increased oxygen free radical-producing activity of polymorphonuclear leukocytes.[11]

Neuroimaging

Three brain imaging techniques have made significant contributions to elucidation of the natural history and pathophysiology of Parkinson's disease, to differential diagnosis of the parkinsonian syndromes, and to the promise of a screening test for patients at risk, perhaps within the foreseeable future. They are:

- Magnetic resonance imaging (MRI)
- Positron emission tomography (PET)
- Single photon emission computed tomography (SPECT).

■ Magnetic Resonance Imaging

The possibility of using MRI to evaluate the severity of pathological changes in the disease has been suggested by the known accumulation of iron in the basal ganglia as well as by the reduced signal from this area with conventional T2 MRI.[12] In a study involving 12 patients with PD and 13 normal, age-matched controls, investigators quantified the effects of paramagnetic centers sequestered inside cellular membranes and derived an index of local tissue iron content for structures of the basal ganglia. They observed a significant increase in iron content in the putamen and pallidum of patients, which correlated with the severity of clinical symptoms. Thus, this novel MRI measurement may provide a noninvasive method of measuring the severity of the pathological changes underlying PD in the future.

■ Positron Emission Tomography

This relatively new imaging technique has contributed significantly to insights into the nigrostriatal dopamine system and its role in the pathophysiology of PD.[13] Clinically, fluorodopa/PET has provided a way to assess the integrity of the striatal dopaminergic terminals. Characteristic reduction of fluorodopa uptake, particularly in the putamen, can be demonstrated in virtually all patients with PD, even in the early stages. Impairment of uptake in an asymptomatic, clinically normal member of a kindred in which five of 10 adult siblings developed apparent PD suggested a subclinical defect in the presynaptic nigrostriatal system.[14]

The density of striatal dopamine (D_2) binding sites is reflected by equilibrium striatal:cerebellar ^{11}C-raclopride (RAC) uptake ratios; PET scans show the receptors to be well preserved in early untreated PD, whereas patients with atypical parkinsonism (striato-nigral degeneration and progressive supranuclear palsy) have a decrease in D_2 density.[15,16] In another long-term study early results in the untreated Parkinson patients were similar. All were treated with L-dopa and dopamine agonists, and 3 to 5 years later, RAC binding was significantly reduced in the putamen and caudate nucleus compared to baseline. This apparent long-term deregulation of striatal D_2 receptor binding may be the result of chronic dopamine therapy or of structural adaptation of the postsynaptic dopaminergic system to the progressive decline of nigrostriatal neurons.

- ### Single Photon Emission Computed Tomography

Ligands have now become available for imaging the pre- and postsynaptic system by SPECT, a valuable contribution to the differential diagnosis between parkinson-plus syndromes and Parkinson's disease, which is a pure presynaptic disorder.[17] Striatal binding of the cocaine derivative [123] beta-CIT, also known as RTI-55, was significantly diminished contralateral to both the clinically affected and unaffected side in hemiparkinsonian patients.[18] Binding was also significantly decreased in comparison to age expected values ranging from 36% in Hoehn and Yahr stage I to 71% in stage V. It is now possible to visualize and quantify the degeneration of nigrostriatal neurons in PD.

Thus, imaging of presynaptic dopamine transporters using this or other new ligands may prove to be useful in early detection of individuals at risk. In fact, SPECT's potential as a screening method for early or even presymptomatic PD seems to have become a practical reality.[17] The technique's potential as an objective method of monitoring the efficacy of new pharmacologic therapies is currently being studied.

The promise of this approach is enhanced by the relative simplicity and lower cost of SPECT compared to the other neuroimaging techniques.

Parkinson's Disease Rating Scales

Clinical evaluation of patients with a disease such as Parkinson's, with its multiple signs and symptoms that differ in presence and intensity among patients, is a complex, often difficult endeavor. Evaluation can be quantitative, with measurements in objective, physical units, or qualitative, using subjective scales to assess symptoms and signs and/or functional disability.[19] Quantitative testing with its often time-consuming methods and expensive or sophisticated equipment, is not generally used to assess and follow patients with Parkinson's disease. Nor is it useful in the evaluation of the large number of patients involved in clinical trials.

Qualitative testing, on the other hand, is relatively rapid and simple and is generally used by neurologists in the staging, evaluation, and following of Parkinson patients. A number of rating scales, with a somewhat standardized core of assessment and a four-point scoring system, have been designed. One of the most widely used, the Unified Parkinson's Disease Rating Scale (UPDRS), assesses 42 items, scored from 0 to 4, to establish individual patients' mental status, activities of daily living, motor function, and complications of therapy (Table 7.7). The UPDRS is often accompanied by a Step-Second Test (Table 7.8) and the Schwab and England Activities of Daily Living Scale (Table 7.9).

TABLE 7.7 — UNIFIED PARKINSON'S DISEASE RATING SCALE (UPDRS)

Mentation, Behavior and Mood

Intellectual Impairment

0= None.

1= Mild. Consistent forgetfulness with partial recollection of events and no other difficulties.

2= Moderate memory loss, with disorientation and moderate difficulty handling complex problems. Mild but definite impairment of function at home with need of occasional prompting.

3= Severe memory loss with disorientation for time and often to place. Severe impairment in handling problems.

4= Severe memory loss with orientation preserved to person only. Unable to make judgements or solve problems. Requires much help with personal care. Cannot be left alone at all.

Thought Disorder (Due to dementia or drug intoxication)

0= None.

1= Vivid dreaming.

2= "Benign" hallucinations with insight retained.

3= Occasional to frequent hallucinations or delusions; without insight; could interfere with daily activities.

4= Persistent hallucinations, delusions, or florid psychosis. Not able to care for self.

Depression

0= Not present.

1= Periods of sadness or guilt greater than normal, never sustained for days or weeks.

2= Sustained depression (1 week or more).

3= Sustained depression with vegetative symptoms (insomnia, anorexia, weight loss, loss of interest).

4= Sustained depression with vegetative symptoms and suicidal thoughts or intent.

Motivation/Initiative

0= Normal.

1= Less assertive than usual, more passive.

2= Loss of initiative or disinterest in elective (non-routine) activities.

3= Loss of initiative or disinterest in day-to-day (routine) activities.

4= Withdrawn, complete loss of motivation.

Activities of Daily Living
(Determine for "On"/"Off")

Speech

0= Normal.
1= Mildly affected; no difficulty being understood.
2= Moderately affected; sometimes asked to repeat statements.
3= Severely affected; frequently asked to repeat statements.
4= Unintelligible most of the time.

Salivation

0= Normal.
1= Slight but definite excess of saliva in mouth; may have night-time drooling.
2= Moderately excessive saliva; may have minimal drooling.
3= Marked excess of saliva with some drooling.
4= Marked drooling, requires constant tissue or handkerchief.

Swallowing

0= Normal.
1= Rare choking.
2= Occasional choking.
3= Requires soft food.
4= Requires NG tube or gastrotomy feeding.

Handwriting

0= Normal.
1= Slightly slow or small.
2= Moderately slow or small; all words are legible.
3= Severely affected; not all words are legible.
4= The majority of words are not legible.

Cutting Food and Handling Utensils

0= Normal.
1= Somewhat slow and clumsy, but no help needed.
2= Can cut most foods, although clumsy and slow; some help needed.
3= Food must be cut by someone, but can still feed slowly.
4= Needs to be fed.

Dressing

0= Normal.
1= Somewhat slow, but no help needed.
2= Occasional assistance with buttoning, getting arms in sleeves.
3= Considerable help required, but can do some things alone.
4= Helpless.

Continued

Hygiene

0= Normal.
1= Somewhat slow, but no help needed.
2= Needs help to shower or bathe; or very slow in hygienic care.
3= Requires assistance for washing, brushing teeth, combing hair, using the toilet.
4= Helpless (foley catheter or other mechanical aids needed).

Turning in Bed and Adjusting Bed Clothes

0= Normal.
1= Somewhat slow and clumsy, but no help needed.
2= Can turn alone or adjust sheets, but with great difficulty.
3= Can initiate movement, but not turn or adjust sheets alone.
4= Helpless.

Falling (Unrelated to Freezing)

0= None.
1= Rare falling.
2= Occasionally falls, less than once per day.
3= Falls an average of once daily.
4= Falls more than once daily.

Freezing When Walking

0= None.
1= Rare freezing when walking; may have start-hesitation.
2= Occasional freezing when walking.
3= Frequent freezing; occasionally falls from freezing.
4= Frequent falls from freezing.

Walking

0= Normal.
1= Mild difficulty; may not swing arms or may tend to drag leg.
2= Moderate difficulty, but requires little or no assistance.
3= Cannot walk at all, even with assistance.

Tremor

0= Absent.
1= Slight and infrequently present.
2= Moderate; bothersome to patient.
3= Severe; interferes with many activities.
4= Marked; interferes with most activities.

Sensory Complaints Related to Parkinsonism

0= None.
1= Occasionally has numbness, tingling, or mild aching.
2= Frequently has numbness, tingling, or aching; not distressing.
3= Frequent painful sensations.
4= Excruciating pain.

Motor Examination
(Determine for "On"/"Off")

Speech

0= Normal.
1= Slight loss of expression, diction and/or volume.
2= Monotone, slurred but understandable; moderately impaired.
3= Marked impairment, difficult to understand.
4= Unintelligible.

Facial Expression

0= Normal.
1= Slight hypomimia, could be normal "poker face."
2= Slight but definitely abnormal diminution of facial expression.
3= Moderate hypomimia; lips parted some of the time.
4= Masked or fixed facies with severe or complete loss of facial expression; lips parted $1/4$ inch or more.

Tremor at Rest

0= Absent.
1= Slight and infrequently present.
2= Mild in amplitude and persistent; or, moderate in amplitude but only intermittently present.
3= Moderate in amplitude and present most of the time.
4= Marked in amplitude and present most of the time.

Action or Postural Tremor of Hands

0= Absent.
1= Slight; present with action.
2= Moderate in amplitude; present with action.
3= Moderate in amplitude with posture holding as well as action.
4= Marked in amplitude; interferes with feeding.

Rigidity (Judged on passive movement of major joints with patient relaxed in sitting position. Cogwheeling to be ignored.)

0= Absent.
1= Slight or detectable only when activated by mirror or other movements.
2= Mild to moderate.
3= Marked, but full range of motion easily achieved.
4= Severe, range of motion achieved with difficulty.

Continued

Finger Taps (Patient taps thumb with index finger in rapid succession with widest amplitude possible, each hand separately.)

0= Normal ($\geq$ 15/5 seconds).
1= Mild slowing and/or reduction in amplitude (11-14/5 seconds).
2= Moderately impaired. Definite and early fatiguing. May have occasional arrests in movement (7-10/5 seconds).
3= Severely impaired. Frequent hesitation in initiating movements or arrests in ongoing movement (3-6/5 seconds).
4= Can barely perform the task (0-2/5 seconds).

Hand Movements (Patient opens and closes hands in rapid succession with widest amplitude possible, each hand separately.)

0= Normal.
1= Mild slowing and/or reduction in amplitude.
2= Moderately impaired. Definite and early fatiguing. May have occasional arrests in movement.
3= Severely impaired. Frequent hesitation in initiating movements or arrests in ongoing movement.
4= Can barely perform the task.

Rapid Alternating Movements of Hands (Pronation-supination movements of hands, vertically or horizontally, with as large an amplitude as possible, both hands simultaneously.)

0= Normal.
1= Mild slowing and/or reduction in amplitude.
2= Moderately impaired. Definite and early fatiguing. May have occasional arrests in movement.
3= Severely impaired. Frequent hesitation in initiating movements or arrests in ongoing movement.
4= Can barely perform the task.

Leg Agility (With knee bent, patient taps heel on ground in rapid succession, picking up entire leg. Amplitude should be about 3 inches.)

0= Normal.
1= Mild slowing and/or reduction in amplitude.
2= Moderately impaired. Definite and early fatiguing. May have occasional arrests in movement.
3= Severely impaired. Frequent hesitation in initiating movements or arrests in ongoing movement.
4= Can barely perform the task.

Rising From Chair (Patient attempts to arise from a straight-back wood or metal chair, with arms folded across chest.)

0= Normal.

1= Slow; or may need more than one attempt.

2= Pushes self up from arms of seat.

3= Tends to fall back and may have to try more than 1 time, but can get up without help.

4= Unable to rise without help.

Posture

0= Normal erect.

1= Not quite erect, slightly stooped posture; could be normal for older person.

2= Moderately stooped posture, definitely abnormal; can be slightly leaning to one side.

3= Severely stooped posture with kyphosis; can be moderately leaning to one side.

4= Marked flexion with extreme abnormality of posture.

Gait

0= Normal.

1= Walks slowly, may shuffle with short steps, but no festina-tion or propulsion.

2= Walks with difficulty, but requires little or no assistance; may have some festination, short steps, or propulsion.

3= Severe disturbance of gait, requiring assistance.

4= Cannot walk at all, even with assistance.

Postural Stability (Response to sudden posterior displacement produced by pull on shoulders while patient is erect, with eyes open and feet slightly apart. Patient is prepared.)

0= Normal.

1= Retropulsion, but recovers unaided.

2= Absence of postural response; would fall if not caught by examiner.

3= Very unstable, tends to lose balance spontaneously.

4= Unable to stand without assistance.

Body Bradykinesia and Hypokinesia (Combining slowness, hesitancy, decreased arm swing, small amplitude, and poverty of movement in general.)

0= None.

1= Minimal slowness, giving movement a deliberate character; could be normal for some persons. Possibly reduced amplitude.

2= Mild degree of slowness and poverty of movement which is definitely abnormal. Alternatively, some reduced amplitude.

3= Moderate slowness, poverty or small amplitude of movement.

4= Marked slowness, poverty or small amplitude of movement.

Complications of Therapy
(In the past week.)

Dyskinesias
Duration: What proportion of the walking day are dyskinesias present? (Historical information)
 0= None.
 1= 1% to 25% of day.
 2= 26% to 50% of day.
 3= 51% to 75% of day.
 4= 76% to 100% of day.

Disability: How disabling are the dyskinesias? (Historical information; may be modified by office examination)
 0= Not disabling.
 1= Mildly disabling.
 2= Moderately disabling.
 3= Severely disabling.
 4= Completely disabled.

Painful Dyskinesias: How painful are the dyskinesias?
 0= No painful dyskinesias.
 1= Slight.
 2= Moderate.
 3= Severe.
 4= Marked.

Presence of Early Morning Dystonia (Historical information)
 0= No
 1= Yes

Clinical Fluctuations
Are any "off" periods predictable as to timing after a dose of medication?
 0= No
 1= Yes

Are any "off" periods unpredictable as to timing after a dose of medication?
 0= No
 1= Yes

Do any of the "off" periods come on suddenly (eg, over a few seconds)?
 0= No
 1= Yes

What proportion of the walking day is the patient "off" on average?
0= None.
1= 1% to 25% of day.
2= 26% to 50% of day.
3= 51% to 75% of day.
4= 76% to 100% of day.

Other Complications

Does the patient have anorexia, nausea, or vomiting?
0= No
1= Yes

Does the patient have any sleep disturbances (eg, insomnia or hypersomnolence)?
0= No
1= Yes

Does the patient have symptomatic orthostasis?
0= No
1= Yes

Record the patient's blood pressure, pulse, and weight on the scoring form.

Modified Hoehn and Yahr Staging

Stage 0   = No signs of disease.
Stage 1   = Unilateral disease.
Stage 1.5 = Unilateral plus axial involvement.
Stage 2   = Bilateral disease, without impairment of balance.
Stage 2.5 = Mild bilateral disease, with recovery on pull test.
Stage 3   = Mild-to-moderate bilateral disease; some postural instability; physically independent.

TABLE 7.8 — STEP-SECOND TEST

- *Steps Score*: number of steps with right foot per round trip of 15 feet out plus 15 feet back
- *Second Score*: number of seconds per round trip of 15 feet out plus 15 feet back
- *Scoring*:
  0 = Not disabling
  1 = Mildly disabling
  2 = Moderately disabling
  3 = Severely disabling
  4 = Completely disabled

REFERENCES

1. Goetz CG, Jankovic J, Koller WC, Lieberman A, Taylor RB, Waters CH. Preclinical disease, differential diagnosis. *Continuum*. 1995;1(4):26-61.

2. Calne DB, Snow BJ, Lee C. Criteria for diagnosing Parkinson's disease. *Ann Neurol*. 1992;32(suppl):S125-S127.

3. Adams RD, Victor M, Ropper AH, eds. *Principles of Neurology*. 6th ed. New York, NY: McGraw-Hill; 1997:1067-1078.

4. Fahn S. Parkinsonism. In: Rowland LP, ed. *Merritt's Textbook of Neurology*. 9th ed. Baltimore, Md: Williams & Wilkins; 1995:713-730.

5. Gouider-Khouja N, Vidailhet M, Bonnet AM, Pichon J, Agid Y. "Pure" striatonigral degeneration and Parkinson's disease: a comparative clinical study. *Mov Disord*. 1995;10:288-294.

6. Colosimo C, Albanese A, Hughes AJ, de Bruin VM, Lees AJ. Some specific clinical features differentiate multiple system atrophy (striatonigral variety) from Parkinson's disease. *Arch Neurol*. 1995;52:294-298.

7. Hubble JP. Drug-induced parkinsonism. In: Watts RL, Koller WC, eds. *Movement Disorders: Neurologic Principles and Practice*. New York, NY: McGraw-Hill; 1997:325-330.

TABLE 7.9 — SCHWAB AND ENGLAND ACTIVITIES OF DAILY LIVING SCALE

100% ...... Completely independent. Able to do all chores without slowness, difficulty, or impairment. Essentially normal. Unaware of any difficulty.

90% ...... Completely independent. Able to do all chores with some degree of slowness, difficulty, and impairment. Might take twice as long. Beginning to be aware of difficulty.

80% ...... Completely independent in most chores. Takes twice as long. Conscious of difficulty and slowness.

70% ...... Not completely independent. More difficulty with some chores than others. Takes 3 to 4 times as long to complete some chores. Must spend a large part of the day with chores.

60% ...... Some dependency. Can do most chores, but exceedingly slowly and with much effort. Makes errors; some chores impossible.

50% ...... More dependent. Help with half the chores, slower, etc. Difficulty with everything.

40% ...... Very dependent. Can assist with all chores, but can do few alone.

30% ...... With effort, now and then does a few chores alone or begins alone. Much help needed.

20% ...... Nothing alone. Can be a slight help with some chores. Severe invalid.

10% ...... Totally dependent, helpless. Complete invalid.

0% ...... Vegetative, functions such as swallowing, bladder, and bowel functions are not functioning. Bedridden.

8. Hughes AJ, Daniel SE, Kilford L, Lees AJ. Accuracy of clinical diagnosis of idiopathic Parkinson's disease: a clinicopathological study of 100 cases. *J Neurol Neurosurg Psychiatry.* 1992;55:181-184.

9. Nagai Y, Ueno S, Saeki Y, Soga F, Hirano M, Yanagihara T. Decrease of the D_3 dopamine receptor mRNA expression in lymphocytes from patients with Parkinson's disease. *Neurology.* 1996;46:791-795.

10. Factor SA, Ortof E, Dentinger MP, Mankes R, Barron KD. Platelet morphology in Parkinson's disease: an electron microscopic study. *J Neurol Sci.* 1994;122:84-89.

11. Kalra J, Rajput AH, Mantha SV, Chaudhary AK, Prasad K. Oxygen free radical producing activity of polymorphonuclear leukocytes in patients with Parkinson's disease. *Mol Cell Biochem.* 1992;112: 181-186.

12. Ye FQ, Allen PS, Martin WR. Basal ganglia iron content in Parkinson's disease measured with magnetic resonance. *Mov Disord.* 1996;11:243-249.

13. Eidelberg D. Positron emission tomography studies in parkinsonism. *Neurol Clin.* 1992;10:421-433.

14. Sawle GV, Wroe SJ, Lees AJ, Brooks DJ, Frackowiak RS. The identification of presymptomatic parkinsonism: clinical and [^{18}F]dopa positron emission tomography studies in an Irish kindred. *Ann Neurol.* 1992;32:609-617.

15. Brooks DJ, Ibanez V, Sawle GV, et al. Striatal D_2 receptor status in patients with Parkinson's disease, striatonigral degeneration, and progressive supranuclear palsy, measured with ^{11}C-raclopride and positron emission tomography. *Ann Neurol.* 1992;31:184-192.

16. Antonini A, Schwarz J, Oertel WH, Pogarell O, Leenders KL. Long-term changes of striatal dopamine D_2 receptors in patients with Parkinson's disease: a study with positron emission tomography and [^{11}C]raclopride. *Mov Disord.* 1997;12: 33-38.

17. Tissingh G, Booij J, Winogrodzka A, van Royen EA, Wolters EC. IBZM- and CIT-SPECT of the dopaminergic system in parkinsonism. *J Neural Transm.* 1997;50(suppl):31-37.

18. Asenbaum S, Brucke T, Pirker W, et al. Imaging of dopamine transporters with iodine-123-beta-CIT and SPECT in Parkinson's disease. *J Nucl Med.* 1997;38:1-6.

19. Martinez-Martin P, Bermejo-Pareja F. Rating scales in Parkinson's disease. In: Jankovic J, Tolosa E, eds. *Parkinson's Disease and Movement Disorders.* Baltimore, Md: Urban & Schwarzenberg; 1988:235-242.

8 Treatment

The pharmacologic/surgical treatment of Parkinson's disease (PD) can be divided into three major conceptual catagories:[1]

- Symptomatic, to improve signs and symptoms of the disease
- Protective, to interfere with the pathophysiologic mechanisms of the disease
- Restorative, to provide new neurons or to stimulate growth and function of remaining cells (see Chapter 11, *Surgery*).

Although the goal of therapy is to reverse the functional disability, abolition of all symptoms and signs is not currently possible even with high doses of medication. Treatment is, therefore, highly individualized (a retired patient may require less control than one who is still working, for example), and the patient as well as the physician plays a major role in therapeutic decisions.

The treatment of PD with levodopa has been called one of the success stories of modern medicine.[2] The precursor of dopamine in the catecholamine synthetic chain, it can be taken orally because it crosses the blood brain barrier, whereas dopamine does not. When first introduced in the 1960s, the new drug's dramatic results in even severely affected Parkinson patients raised the hope that all neurodegenerative diseases might be treated with replacement of depleted transmitters.[3] But complications of chronic therapy soon became apparent, superimposing upon the disease-related problems an additional burden of motor fluctuations (the "on-off" reaction), dyskinesias, and visual hallucinations.

Although levodopa has remained the most effective drug available for the relief of symptoms in PD, five additional and distinctly different pharmacologic advances during the last 3 decades have significantly augmented the antiparkinson armamentarium:

- Carbidopa, an inhibitor of dopa decarboxylase, which, combined with levodopa, reduces peripheral decarboxylation of levodopa to dopamine
- Controlled release carbidopa/levodopa to prolong levodopa's 90-minute half-life
- Dopamine agonists, sometimes used as pharmacologically active substitutes for carbidopa/levodopa in early disease and to provide supplementation in later stages
- Inhibitors of catechol-0-methyltransferase (COMT) to increase the amount of levodopa crossing the blood-brain barrier
- Monoamine oxidase type B (MAO-B) inhibitors to slow dopamine's metabolic breakdown.

The initial decision in the management of PD is whether any pharmacotherapy is needed.[4] There is no conclusive evidence that treatment is helpful before symptoms start to affect the patient's life. In fact, early-stage disease may be better left untreated if it does not limit motor function. Eventually PD progresses, however, and symptomatic treatment becomes necessary. The decision is usually made on the basis of how symptoms are affecting individual patients, whether they interfere with a job or with the ability to handle domestic, financial, or social affairs. An algorithm for the progressive treatment of PD is seen in Figure 8.1.[5]

Once patient and physician have decided to go ahead with treatment, the choice is whether to introduce levodopa or another antiparkinsonian agent. All patients are likely to develop complications associated

FIGURE 8.1 — THERAPEUTIC ALGORITHM FOR MANAGEMENT OF PARKINSON'S DISEASE

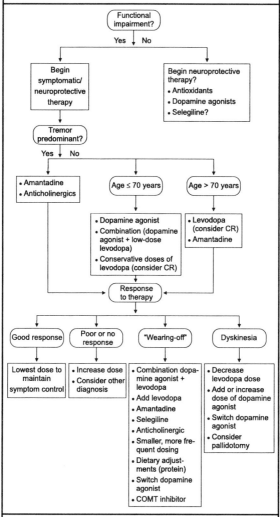

Abbreviations: COMT, catechol-O-methyltransferase; CR, controlled release.

Adapted from: Stern MB. *Neurology*. 1997;49(1 suppl 1):S2-S9.

with long-term use of levodopa. Younger patients, in particular, are more likely to show response fluctuations, so other antiparkinsonian drugs should be considered first to delay the introduction of levodopa.

Levodopa therapy is appropriate if the patient's symptoms are starting to interfere with his or her activities. Patients with mild symptoms may be treated in other ways. Choices include:

- Deferring symptomatic medications until it seems appropriate to start levodopa therapy
- Introducing selegiline for its possible neuroprotective benefit
- Initiating treatment with an anticholinergic drug, amantadine, or a dopamine agonist agent.

Dosage and administration data for the antiparkinson agents are summarized in Table 8.1.

Anticholinergics

Because of the relative sparing of the cholinergic system in PD, coupled with a marked depletion of dopamine, the acetylcholine-dopamine balance in the striatum of PD is tilted in favor of the cholinergic pathways. Not surprisingly, therefore, the symptoms of PD are responsive to anticholinergic agents, which antagonize the cholinergic neurons disinhibited by the loss of dopaminergic neurons.

Anticholinergic agents, the oldest class of drugs used in the treatment of PD, can still be helpful. They are generally thought to be effective for the symptoms of tremor, although rigidity and bradykinesia are not much altered. (However, the response of tremor to anticholinergics as well as to other drugs is highly variable.) And, in some cases, they may be useful adjuvants to levodopa therapy, particularly in patients with motor fluctuations.

TABLE 8.1 — ANTIPARKINSON AGENTS

Generic (Trade) Name	Recommended Dosage	Comments
Anticholinergics	—	Effective for tremor (variably). Use with caution in elderly.
Benztropine (Cogentin)	Initiate: 0.5-1 mg/d at bedtime; can increase to 4-6 mg/d in divided doses.	—
Procyclidine (Kemadrin)	Initiate: 2.5 mg, tid, after meals; increase to 5 mg, tid or qid.	—
Trihexyphenidyl (Artane)	Initiate: First day, 1 mg at mealtime; increase 2 mg/d for 3-5 days to 6 mg/d, tid, at mealtimes.	—
Dopamine Agonists	—	Most effective drugs after levodopa. May be used as monotherapy.
Bromocriptine (Parlodel)	Initiate: ½ of 2.5 mg tablet with meals, bid; increase 2.5 mg/d q 14-28 days to 5-15 mg/d.	—

Continued

8

Generic (Trade) Name	Recommended Dosage	Comments
Dopamine Agonists (cont.)		
Pergolide (Permax)	Initiate: 0.05 mg/d for 2 days; increase 0.10 or 0.15 mg/d q third day for 12 days; increase 0.25 mg/d to 3 mg/d, tid.	Longer duration and less expensive than bromocriptine.
Pramipexole (Mirapex)	Initiate: 0.125 mg, tid; increase q 5-7 days to 3 mg or 4.5 mg/d, tid. (See Table 8.2)	Indicated for both monotherapy and as adjunct to levodopa. Nonergoline, therefore no ergot-related side effects.
Ropinirole (Requip)	Initiate: 0.25 mg/d, tid; increase weekly by 0.25 mg/d, tid, to maximum of 8 mg/d, tid. (See Table 8.3)	Indicated for both monotherapy and as adjunct to levodopa. Superior to bromocriptine, equal to levodopa as monotherapy in early-stage disease. Nonergoline, therefore no ergot-related side effects.
Levodopa		
Carbidopa/Levodopa	Initiate: ½ of 25/100 tablet, bid, after a meal; increase by ½ tablet/d, q 4-7 days.	"Gold standard" of parkinsonian therapy. Timing of initiation controversial.
Carbidopa/Levodopa Controlled-Release	Initiate: 25/100 tablet or 50/200 tablet, bid.	Effective for sleep. Just as likely to produce motor fluctuations as regular Sinemet.

COMT Inhibitor		
Tolcapone (Tasmar)	100 mg or 200 mg, tid, q 6 h.	Adjunct to levodopa.
Entacapone (Comtan)*	200 mg with each dose of levodopa.	Adjunct to levodopa.
Other		
Amantadine (Symmetrel)	As monotherapy or in combination: 100-200 mg/d.	Global improvement of 20% to 40% in 66% of patients; minimal effect on tremor. Loss of efficacy within 6-8 months. Acts synergistically with levodopa.
Selegiline (Eldepryl)	5 mg at breakfast and lunch; 5 mg/d may be effective in some patients.	Delays the need for levodopa. Prolongs levodopa's symptomatic benefits. May be neuroprotective.
Abbreviations: COMT, catechol-O-methyltransferase.		
* Investigational in the United States.		

8

■ Dosage and Administration

- Trihexyphenidyl (Artane)
  - Initiate with 1 mg at mealtime
  - Increase 2 mg/day for 3 to 5 days to 6 mg/day, tid, at mealtimes
- Benztropine (Cogentin)
  - Initiate with 0.5 mg to 1 mg at bedtime
  - Can increase to 4 mg to 6 mg/day if needed, bid or qid
- Procyclidine (Kemadrin)
  - Initiate with 2.5 mg, tid, after meals
  - Increase to 5 mg/day, tid or qid.

These drugs have a number of side effects, including:

- Dry mouth
- Narrow-angle glaucoma
- Constipation
- Urinary retention
- Memory impairment
- Confusion, hallucinations.

The anticholinergics should be used with caution if at all in the elderly since they have a poor therapeutic index and high toxicity.

Amantadine (Symmetrel)

Patients whose early symptoms do not respond to anticholinergics may benefit from substitution by or addition of amantadine. An antiviral agent found to have an antiparkinsonian effect as well, amantadine's precise mechanism of action remains to be defined. However, it releases dopamine from peripheral neuronal storage sites of animals who have received infusions of the transmitters, suggesting it might exert a similar action on the residual, intact dopaminergic terminals in the striatum of parkinsonian patients.[6] Among the other reported actions are:

- Release of dopamine from central neurons
- Delay of dopamine uptake by neural cells
- Blockade of N-methyl-D-aspartate (NMDA) receptors[7]
- Anticholinergic effects.

Amantadine reportedly results in 20% to 40% global improvement in two thirds of patients when given as monotherapy for early, minor symptoms. It seems to have only a minimal effect on tremor and the development of tolerance in some instances.[6]

Amantadine is also effective in later stages of the disease; patients who are obtaining near-maximal or waning benefits from levodopa usually derive some additional benefit because of the additive actions of the two drugs.[6]

8

■ Dosage and Administration

As monotherapy or in combination with other antiparkinson drugs:

- 100 mg bid
- If response is diminished after a few months, efficacy may be regained by increase to 300 mg/day after a few-weeks holiday.

Compared with the anticholinergic agents, amantadine is relatively free of side effects, which may include:

- Hallucinations
- Leg edema
- Livedo reticularis (mottled skin) on legs.

Selegiline (Eldepryl)

An irreversible inhibitor of MAO-B, an enzyme associated with the outer membrane of mitochondria, selegiline, or L-deprenyl, is indicated as an adjunct to carbidopa/levodopa (see *Carbidopa/Levodopa*) for patients who exhibit deterioration in response to levodopa.[5] Selegiline has been shown to prolong the symptomatic benefit of levodopa.

Given some evidence that selegiline may have some neuroprotective effect, a large, multicenter trial, the Deprenyl and Tocopherol Antioxidant Therapy of Parkinsonism (DATATOP), by the Parkinson Study Group, was designed to determine whether the two agents (deprenyl and tocopherol) could delay the need for levodopa therapy in newly diagnosed patients.[8] The basis for the study, which involved 800 patients, was the finding that inhibition of MAO-B prevented toxin methyl phenyl tetrahydropyridine (MPTP)-induced parkinsonism in primates. According to preliminary results of the DATATOP study, the risk of reaching the end point (onset of disability requiring levodopa) was reduced by 57% for patients receiving deprenyl.

A symptomatic effect was suggested by improvement of motor scores after the initiation of deprenyl and deterioration of scores on its withdrawal. However, statistically reduced disability compared to placebo was found even among deprenyl patients who initially had no improvement in motor scores, suggesting a neuroprotective effect.

In a second study by the same group of investigators, 310 of the patients who did not reach the end point received deprenyl.[9] The original blinding as to those who did or did not receive the drug initially was maintained. Thus, if those who had received the drug initially showed superior and sustained benefit from its reinitiation compared to those not previously treated with deprenyl, the drug probably had a neuroprotective effect. However, 189 patients who had been assigned to deprenyl originally reached the end point of disability faster than the 121 who had not been assigned to it. The conclusion, that the initial advantages of deprenyl were not sustained, was not definitive, however, primarily because the deprenyl patients had more severe impairment at baseline, because of the 2-month interruption of therapy, and the many problems associated with the interpretation of open-label trials.[10]

The issue of neuroprotection with deprenyl was then addressed in a 14-month, prospective, randomized, double-blind study in which patients who were untreated at baseline received deprenyl and levodopa.[11] Deprenyl was withdrawn 2 months and levodopa 7 to 14 days before the final visit. Placebo-treated patients deteriorated by 5.8 points on the Unified Parkinson's Disease Rating Scale (UPDRS), whereas those who received deprenyl changed by only 0.4 points, clear evidence that the drug prevents deterioration in clinical scores in patients with early PD.[10]

Although these observed effects are more readily explained by a neuroprotective than symptomatic action, other explanations are also possible. For example, recent reports suggest that deprenyl's mechanism of action may involve pathways other than MAO-B inhibition, based on finding that:

- Deprenyl alters the expression of a number of mRNAs or proteins in nerve and glial cells, and these alterations are:
  - The result of a selective action on transcription
  - Accompanied by a decrease in DNA fragmentation characteristic of apoptosis[12]
- In doses that do not inhibit MAO-B, deprenyl limits free radical formation and prevents nigral damage due to the direct administration of methyl phenylpyridinium ion (MPP+).[12-14]

Despite some strong evidence of selegiline's possible neuroprotective effect, however, it remains to be proven.[10] Furthermore, if the drug does influence disease progression, it seems only to mildly slow the course; progression is not halted.[15]

■ Selegiline Monotherapy

All things considered, once the diagnosis of PD is made, selegiline is a reasonable medication for some patients with minor nondisabling symptoms. It serves as a hedge against both the major issues of controversy:[15]

- The initial DATATOP and more recent study results suggesting selegiline's neuroprotective effects
- The oxidant stress hypothesis, which predicts that levodopa treatment toxicity will be reduced by selegiline inhibition of MAO-B oxidation of dopamine.

Appropriate candidates for selegiline monotherapy are:

- Early-stage patients without disabling symptoms
- Young patients ($\leq$ 65 years of age).

Higher doses provide no additional therapeutic advantages, and doses above 30 mg/day also inhibit monoamine oxidase type A (MAO-A), with the potential for hypertensive crisis (cheese effect). The cheese effect is not a concern with conventional dosage, however; thus, no dietary modifications are necessary.

According to the DATATOP trials, selegiline monotherapy is typically well tolerated, at least in early Parkinson patients.[8,9] Cognitively impaired patients probably should not be prescribed the drug since it could lead to cognitive decompensation and psychosis.

■ **Selegiline as Adjunctive Therapy**

An open, long-term, prospective, randomized trial comparing levodopa (with the dopa decarboxylase inhibitor benserazide) and the combination of levodopa/benserazide and selegiline in early, mild PD was launched by the United Kingdom's Parkinson's Research Group in 1985.[16] Patients were evaluated at baseline, then every 3 to 4 months, with interim analyses once a year.

The interim 3-year report indicated that both treatments led to improvement in baseline disabilities after 1 year of continuous treatment but that functional disability and physical signs had deteriorated after 3 years. No significant difference in mortality was seen at that time.

However, after an average 5.6 years, the difference in survival in the two treatment groups was significant (Figure 8.2). Mortality was about 60% higher in patients given combined treatment than in those given levodopa alone. Disability scores were slightly, nonsignificantly, higher in the levodopa monotherapy group, but severe motor complications were more frequent in patients given combined therapy.

This is the first study to report such a finding. Analysis of mortality in other, ongoing studies will be needed to see whether it can be corroborated.

■ **Dosage and Administration**
- 10 mg/day, 5 mg at breakfast and lunch
- 5 mg/day may be effective in some patients.

Vitamin E (Tocopherol)

Another debate, whether high intake of antioxidants decreases the risk of PD, is based on an early (unrandomized, uncontrolled) study of vitamin E supplements in patients who develop PD before the usual age of onset.[2] Patients who received vitamin E

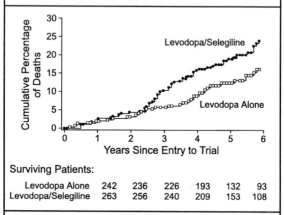

FIGURE 8.2 — COMPARATIVE MORTALITY IN PATIENTS TREATED WITH LEVODOPA ALONE AND WITH LEVODOPA AND SELEGILINE

Surviving Patients:

Levodopa Alone	242	236	226	193	132	93
Levodopa/Selegiline	263	256	240	209	153	108

The cumulative percentage of deaths among patients treated with dopa decarboxylase inhibitor/levodopa alone appears to be significantly lower than among those who received both the levodopa preparation and selegiline in this Kaplan-Meier estimate.

Adapted from: Lees AJ. *BMJ*. 1995;311:1602-1607.

3200 IU daily survived a mean 2.5 years longer without levodopa than those who received no vitamin E supplementation. The debate was joined when DATATOP data failed to reproduce these results, albeit with only 2000 IU of vitamin E per day.

Epidemiologic data have suggested that patients with PD had consumed less vitamin E in the premorbid period, and those who had self-supplemented with vitamin E had a more benign clinical course than those who did not. According to a later report, however, PD brains are not deficient in vitamin E.

The most recent pro report comes from a community-based study in which 5,342 independently living individuals between 55 and 95 years of age, 31 with PD, were administered a semiquantitative food frequency questionnaire.[17] The investigators concluded that a high intake of dietary vitamin E may protect against the occurrence of PD.

Dopamine Agonists

Because they bypass the failing nigrostriatal pathway to directly stimulate receptors in the normal striatum, dopamine agonist agents, unlike levodopa, do not require conversion and storage. They are the most effective class of drugs for PD after levodopa. In early disease, they may be as beneficial as levodopa and provide an effective treatment strategy, delaying the need for levodopa. Four dopamine agonists are currently available:

- Bromocriptine (Parlodel)
- Pergolide (Permax)
- Pramipexole (Mirapex)
- Ropinirole (Requip).

There is clear preclinical evidence indicating that dopamine agonists with a long half-life are associated with less risk of developing dyskinesia than levodopa. There is recent compelling evidence with the newer dopamine agonists that levodopa can be delayed for a number of years. Therefore, I recommend the use of these compounds prior to levodopa initiation in early disease to avoid or delay the production of dyskinesia.

The basis for the development of dyskinesia appears to depend on disease severity and the half-life of the dopaminergic agent. Patients who have mild disease do not develop dyskinesia with either levodopa or dopamine agonists, presumably because they still have enough dopamine terminals to regulate dopamine release and provide postsynaptic dopamine receptors with relatively physiologic dopaminergic stimulation. In more advanced disease, there are not enough dopamine terminals to regulate dopamine release, resulting in fluctuations in striatal levodopa. The resulting exposure of striatal receptors to alternating high and low concentrations of dopamine seems to induce the postsynaptic changes that lead to the development of dyskinesia and motor complications. Dopamine agonists that act directly on the dopamine receptor have the potential to provide longer, more physiologic stimulation of receptors and prevent development of such changes. Unlike levodopa, with its brief half-life of 60 to 90 minutes, dopamine agonists with half-lives of more than 5 to 6 hours are not as associated with the development of dyskinesias.

Initial monotherapy may be more useful in younger patients, who are more prone to the early development of levodopa-related clinical fluctuations and who will have to be treated for a longer time than those with older onset.[18]

The question of whether early combination therapy with lower-dose levodopa and dopamine agonist will delay disability has no definitive answer. The use of the dopamine agonists to prolong the symptomatic benefit of levodopa in patients with advanced, fluctuating disease is discussed in Chapter 9, *Complications of Parkinson's Disease and its Therapy.*

■ Bromocriptine (Parlodel)

An ergot alkaloid with potent D_2 agonist effects, bromocriptine is approved as adjunctive therapy to carbidopa/levodopa for patients who develop tolerance to levodopa and end-of-dose failure.[6]

Dosage and Administration
- Initial dose, ½ of 2.5 mg tablet bid with meals
- Increase every 14 to 28 days by 2.5 mg/day
- Therapeutic dose is usually 5 mg to 7.5 mg/day (range 2.5 mg to 15 mg/day).

The addition of bromocriptine may permit reduction in the maintenance dose of levodopa.

The most common side effects of bromocriptine are:

- Nausea
- Dyskinesia
- Hallucinations
- Confusion
- Postural hypotension.

A variety of bromocriptine dosage regimens have been used as monotherapy in the treatment of early or mild Parkinson disease.[1] In the usual doses prescribed in the United States and Canada, up to 30 mg/day, only one third of patients can be maintained on monotherapy for more than 1 year. In higher doses, monotherapy can be maintained for 3 to 5 years. Adverse reactions have been minimal. Mental changes can occur but dyskinesias are rarely a problem.

According to product labeling, however, data are insufficient to evaluate potential benefit from treating newly diagnosed PD patients with bromocriptine.[17] Studies have shown significantly more adverse reactions in bromocriptine-treated than in carbidopa/levodopa-treated patients.

■ Pergolide (Permax)

Also an ergot derivative, pergolide stimulates both D_1 and D_2 dopamine receptors. Like bromocriptine, it is indicated as adjunctive treatment with carbidopa/levodopa.

Pergolide has only infrequently been studied in the treatment of early PD.[1] In three open-label, randomized trials of its efficacy and safety:[18]

- As monotherapy in 86 untreated patients, pergolide resulted in marked or moderate improvement in 47.5% and mild improvement in 32%.

- In a short-term, double-blind trial comparing the efficacy of pergolide with that of bromocriptine in both *de novo* and add-on groups:
  - In *de novo* patients, the agonist agents demonstrated similar efficacy
  - Significantly more levodopa-treated patients in the pergolide group showed marked or moderate improvement
- In a long-term study of the levodopa-pergolide combination:
  - 151 of 314 patients remained in the study for 3 years, 127 for 4 years, with maintenance of initial improvement
  - In 18 of 62 *de novo* patients, initial improvement was maintained for up to 3 years.

Pergolide has a longer duration of effect than bromocriptine.

Dosage and Administration
- Initiate with 0.05 mg/day for first 2 days
- Increase gradually by 0.10 or 0.15 mg/day every third day over next 12 days
- Increase by 0.25 mg/day every third day to optimal dose
- Therapeutic dose range, 0.75 mg to 3 mg/day in divided doses, tid.

Such gradual titration is important given the approximately 10% of patients in clinical trials who experienced symptomatic, orthostatic, and/or sustained hypotension.

The other most commonly seen side effects of pergolide are:
- Dyskinesia
- Hallucinations
- Somnolence
- Insomnia

- Nausea
- Constipation
- Diarrhea
- Dyspepsia.

■ Pramipexole (Mirapex)

Pramipexole is a nonergot benzothiazole derivative. It is a potent dopamine benzothiazole agonist that binds to the D_3 receptor subtype of the D_2 receptor class.[19] The indication for pramipexole is somewhat broader than that for the ergot derivatives bromocriptine and pergolide for the treatment of the signs and symptoms of PD.

Pramipexole as Monotherapy

In studies of the drug's efficacy in early disease it was found to be safe and effective as short-term monotherapy. A 9-week trial in 55 patients not yet taking levodopa found statistically significant improvement in patients receiving pramipexole as compared to placebo on part II (activities of daily living) of the UPDRS.[20]

All subjects in both the pramipexole and placebo groups experienced one or more episodes of asymptomatic postural hypotension; no significant difference was found between the two groups in number of subjects experiencing symptomatic orthostatic hypertension.

A second, 24-week multicenter, randomized, double-blind trial involved 335 early-stage patients not receiving levodopa.[21] Each was titrated to his or her maximally well-tolerated dose of study medication for up to 7 weeks before the 6-month follow-up. Results included:

- Pramipexole significantly reduced the severity of PD as measured by decreases in parts II (activities of daily living) and III (motor signs) of the UPDRS

- Only nausea, constipation, and insomnia had a 10% higher incidence rate in pramipexole compared with placebo patients
- No clinically significant changes were noted in blood pressure or pulse rate.

Finally, a 10-week, randomized, dose ranging (1.5 to 6.0 mg/day) trial, which involved 264 patients who had not received levodopa, also found pramipexole to be safe and effective as short-term monotherapy.[22] Findings were:
- A 20% improvement in total UPDRS scores, largely motor benefits, similar for all dosages
- Evidence that treatment effects were more pronounced in subjects with worse UPDRS scores at baseline.

In this study, somnolence was reported with greater frequency in the pramipexole group.

Pramipexole as Adjunctive Therapy

Pramipexole's role as adjunctive therapy in advanced PD has been addressed in two clinical trials. One trial, an 11-week, single-blind parallel group, placebo-controlled trial involving 24 patients with motor fluctuations found:[23]
- A significant improvement in "off" time
- A reduction of 30% in levodopa dose
- Dyskinesia worsened in half the patients.

A second study of pramipexole as adjunct was conducted in two parts: a 32-week, double-blind, placebo-controlled, parallel-group study, followed by an open-label extension trial (results not available at this writing).[24] Of 360 patients with advanced disease and "wearing-off" phenomenon, 181 were randomized to pramipexole, 179 to placebo (0.375 mg to 4.5 mg/day, increased daily to maximal tolerated or stable improvement).

The primary end points were change from baseline to final maintenance visit of the average of the "on" and "off" ratings for:

- UPDRS part II (activities of daily living)
- UPDRS part III (parkinsonian motor signs).

A number of secondary end points included changes from baseline to final visit in Schwab and England Disability Scale, Hoehn and Yahr stage, and patient diaries.

Patients were followed for 6 months. Compared to placebo, pramipexole, at a maximal daily dosage of 4.5 mg:

- Improved activities of daily living as determined by UPDRS part II, assessed in the "on" and "off" periods and averaged
- Improved motor function as determined by UPDRS part III motor evaluation, assessed in the "on" period
- An overall statistically significant decrease in the severity of the "off" periods (Figure 8.3)
- A 27% reduction in the dosage of levodopa.

The magnitude of improvement in activities of daily living (21%), motor evaluation (25%), and time in the "off" period (31%) compared favorably with that of other dopamine agonists. Central nervous system adverse events were also similar. Gastrointestinal and cardiovascular side effects were less frequent.

The most recently reported multicenter, double-blind, placebo-controlled, randomized trial involved 246 patients with wearing-off (Hoehn and Yahr stage II to IV during "on" times).[25] It included three phases:

- Dose escalation
- Six months' maintenance
- Dose reduction.

FIGURE 8.3 — "OFF" PERIODS ASSOCIATED WITH PRAMIPEXOLE AND PLACEBO

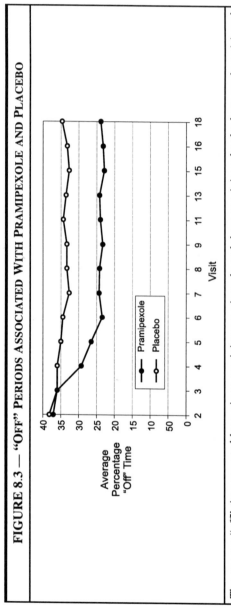

The percent "off" time reported by patients receiving pramipexole and those receiving placebo between last visit and baseline shows a statistically significant decrease in favor of pramipexole.

Adapted from: Lieberman A, et al. *Neurology*. 1997;49:162-168.

A bromocriptine treatment group was included to enable comparisons between bromocriptine and placebo groups, but the study was not planned to show statistical differences between pramipexole and bromocriptine.

Up to 4.5 mg/day of pramipexole and 30 mg of bromocriptine were used. Primary end points were changes in UPDRS parts II and III. Results included:

- UPDRS part II improvements of 26.7% for pramipexole, 14% for bromocriptine, 4.8% for placebo
- No major differences in safety data
- Comparison of global clinical assessment of efficacy between active treatment groups showed a trend to significance in favor of pramipexole
- More reports of dyskinesia and nausea in both treatment groups compared to placebo.

Dosage and Administration

Pramipexole should be titrated gradually to achieve a maximum therapeutic effect balanced against the principal side effects of dyskinesia, hallucinations, somnolence, and dry mouth. For initial treatment:

- Increase gradually from a starting dose of 0.125 mg/day, tid
- Should not be increased more frequently than every 5 to 7 days.

A suggested ascending dosage schedule, which was used in clinical studies, is shown in Table 8.2. There are dosing recommendations for patients with renal impairment which involve reducing the frequency and thus total maximum daily dose.

There is strong evidence that pramipexole is an excellent medication for early PD. Its role in more

TABLE 8.2 — ASCENDING DOSAGE SCHEDULE FOR PRAMIPEXOLE (MIRAPEX)		
Week	Dosage (mg)	Total Daily Dose (mg)
1	0.125 tid	0.375
2	0.25 tid	0.75
3	0.5 tid	1.5
4	0.75 tid	2.25
5	1.0 tid	3.0
6	1.25 tid	3.75
7	1.5 tid	4.5

advanced disease seems to be similar to that seen with other dopamine agonists.

Adverse experiences with pramipexole were found to be similar to those of other dopamine agonists, although symptomatic orthostatic hypotension was uncommon.

■ Ropinirole (Requip)

Ropinirole has a novel, nonergoline structure closely based on that of dopamine.[26] This chemical structure has the potential to maintain a structure-activity relationship similar to that of dopamine and other effective dopamine agonists without producing ergot-related adverse effects. Ropinirole has been shown to exert a presynaptic effect via stimulation of dopamine D_2 and D_3 receptors, binding with a higher affinity to D_3 receptors.

Ropinirole as Monotherapy

Ropinirole has been assessed as monotherapy in early disease in three double-blind, randomized, controlled, multicenter trials:[27]

- A 6-month placebo-controlled trial involving 241 patients[28]

- An ongoing 5-year levodopa-controlled study of 268 patients[29]
- A 3-year bromocriptine-controlled trial (prospectively stratified for selegiline use) of 335 patients.[30,31]

Patients enrolled in these studies had early PD, had not been treated with levodopa (or treated for no more than 6 weeks) and, in the investigators' opinion, were in need of dopaminergic therapy. Ropinirole or comparator were titrated according to patient response, and the principal measure of efficacy was the UPDRS motor score, including:

- Percentage of patients who achieved a greater than 30% reduction in the score
- Percentage who were "improved" according to a 7-point Clinical Global Impression (CGI) scale
- Percentage of patients who required levodopa rescue therapy during the study.

To summarize the efficacy of ropinirole as monotherapy during the first 6 months of treatment of early PD:

- Patients on ropinirole showed statistically significant improvement in the UPDRS motor scores (24% reduction) compared to placebo (3% worsening).
- Ropinirole was as effective as levodopa in early disease[32] (see Figure 8.4).
- Ropinirole was significantly superior to bromocriptine in patients not receiving selegiline (Figure 8.5). Three-year data show 60% of patients completing the study still on ropinirole monotherapy.

In a 6-month extension study of the first (241 patients) of the three trials, 147 of the patients were con-

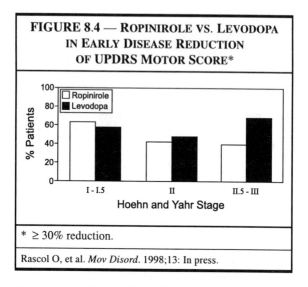

FIGURE 8.4 — ROPINIROLE VS. LEVODOPA IN EARLY DISEASE REDUCTION OF UPDRS MOTOR SCORE*

* ≥ 30% reduction.

Rascol O, et al. *Mov Disord*. 1998;13: In press.

tinued on double-blind medication without interruption.[33] Of those receiving ropinirole, 44% remained on ropinirole alone without addition of levodopa compared to 22.4% of placebo patients. The ropinirole group also experienced a 30% reduction in UPDRS motor score as well as significant improvement on the CGI scale (Figure 8.6). Ropinirole continued to be well tolerated, with only three patients withdrawing because of adverse experiences. Although all three clinical trials have been designed to test ropinirole's efficacy as early therapy and to determine its ability to replace or significantly delay the need for levodopa, only 12-month results have been formally reported. Three-year data show a small percentage of patients experience dyskinesia (3% to 4%) on dopamine agonist monotherapy.

Ropinirole as Adjunctive Therapy

As an adjunct to levodopa in later stage patients not adequately controlled with levodopa, ropinirole has been studied in four controlled clinical studies:[27]

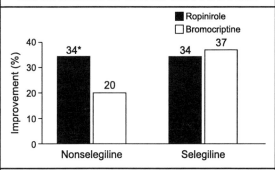

FIGURE 8.5 — ROPINIROLE AND BROMOCRIPTINE AS MONOTHERAPY: COMPARATIVE IMPROVEMENT IN UPDRS MOTOR SCORE

* Significantly different from bromocriptine.

On the Unified Parkinson's Disease Rating Scale (UPDRS) motor score, ropinirole alone, without selegiline, was significantly superior to bromocriptine alone in patients with early Parkinson's disease who had not been treated with levodopa (or treated no more than 6 weeks).

Adapted from: Korczyn AD, et al. *Mov Disord.* 1998;13:In press.

- A 3-month, placebo-controlled trial in 46 patients experiencing mild-to-moderate fluctuations[34]
- A placebo-controlled study of 68 patients with motor fluctuations[27]
- A 6-month, placebo-controlled study of 148 patients not optimally controlled by levodopa (which could be decreased during trial)
- A 6-month study comparing ropinirole and bromocriptine in 555 patients.[27]

Results of these studies show that when ropinirole is used as an adjunct to levodopa in patients with advanced PD and motor fluctuations:[27]

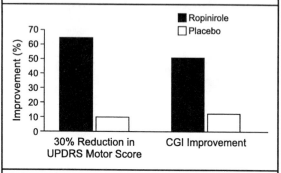

FIGURE 8.6 — ROPINIROLE AND PLACEBO: 12-MONTH UPDRS AND CGI RESULTS

Patients taking ropinirole alone for the symptoms of early Parkinson's disease showed significant improvement in both Unified Parkinson's Disease Rating Scale (UPDRS) motor score and on the blinded investigators' Clinical Global Impression (CGI) scale.

Adapted from: Kreider MS, et al. *Neurology.* 1997;48:A269. Abstract.

- Ropinirole reduces awake time spent "off" by an average of 2 to 3 hours when levodopa is not reduced.
- The addition of ropinirole to levodopa allows an average reduction in daily levodopa dose of 20% once a therapeutic dose of the agonist is reached.
- Ropinirole is superior to placebo in generating significant improvement in patients with motor fluctuations.
- Results comparing ropinirole and bromocriptine as adjunctive treatment are unclear.

In monotherapy studies, adverse events are mostly in the range of what is expected of a dopamine agonist. Nausea was the most common but was generally well-tolerated and disappeared over time. (Domperidone, where available, may reduce the nausea.) In adjunct trials, nausea occurred at a much lower rate.

Dizziness, postural hypotension, and syncope were also observed in PD patients and were seen in the ropinirole group as well as in the active comparator groups.

Somnolence was seen in some patients. The incidence of psychiatric episodes was low in the early short-term therapy studies with no clear differences between confusion and hallucinations compared to levodopa or bromocriptine.

Dosage and Administration

Whether ropinirole is to be used as monotherapy or as an adjunct to levodopa:

- Initiate therapy with 0.25 mg, tid
- Increase in weekly increments (see Table 8.3)
- Patients may feel benefit by week 4 (1.0 mg, tid)
- Dosage may be increased in weekly increments to a maximum dose of 8 mg, tid
- The titration schedule may be slower, but faster increases are not recommended.

TABLE 8.3 — ASCENDING DOSAGE SCHEDULE FOR ROPINIROLE (REQUIP)		
Week	**Dosage (mg)**	**Total Daily Dose (mg)**
1	0.25 tid	0.75 mg
2	0.5 mg tid	1.5 mg
3	0.75 mg tid	2.25 mg
4	1.0 mg tid	3.0 mg
Doses greater than 24 mg/day have not been tested in clinical trials.		

In patients with moderate renal impairment (creatinine clearance, 30 mL to 50 mL/min), no dosage adjustment of ropinirole is necessary. Its use in severe renal impairment has not been studied.

Thus, there is strong evidence that ropinirole is an excellent medicine in early PD. It may substitute for levodopa for several years. As adjunct to levodopa in later disease, it is beneficial in ameliorating wearing-off phenomenon.

COMT Inhibitors

Although the addition of carbidopa to levodopa increases the amount of the drug available to cross the blood-brain barrier, most levodopa is then metabolized in the gut and liver (first-pass metabolism) by catechol-O-methyltransferase (COMT) to an inactive metabolite, 3-O-methyldopa (3-OMD). The COMT inhibitory agents, tolcapone and entacapone, prevent this breakdown, thus prolonging the half-life of levodopa and increasing its transport into the brain to raise dopamine levels.

■ Tolcapone (Tasmar)

A potent inhibitor of both peripheral and central COMT, tolcapone has been investigated as adjunctive therapy with carbidopa/levodopa for both early, mild PD and for advanced disease, complicated by levodopa-related motor fluctuations.

Tolcapone as Adjunct to Levodopa

Most clinical trials of tolcapone have involved patients with motor fluctuations. In one of the first, a multicenter, double-blind, placebo-controlled study, 151 patients from 12 centers were studied before and after 6 weeks of tolcapone (50 mg, 100 mg, or 400 mg, tid).[35] Clinical evaluations lasting 10 hours were performed on days 1 and 42, using the UPDRS subscale and "on/off" and dyskinesia assessments every 30 minutes.

Primary outcome measures were changes in "off" time and in the area under the curve (AUC) for UPDRS scores during the two 10-hour assessments. Among the secondary outcome measures were patient diary evaluation of "on/off" time and change in intake frequency and total daily dose of levodopa.

Treatment with tolcapone resulted in a clinically significant reduction of "off" time, increase in "on" time (Figure 8.7), and reduction in the requirement for levodopa. Specific results, according to dosage, included:

- A 47% decrease in "off" time with the 400-mg dose (not significantly different from 50-mg and 200-mg doses)
- Improvement in "on" time was substantially higher for the 200-mg dose (86%) compared to the 50-mg (33%) and 400-mg (40%) doses.
- UPDRS motor AUC was significantly reduced, with the 200-mg dose offering the greatest reduction (not significantly different from 400-mg dose)
- A significant decrease in number of daily doses of carbidopa/levodopa seen at the 200-mg and 400-mg doses, representing a mean reduction of approximately 1½ doses a day (200-mg dose associated with greatest total daily dosage reduction).

Like other agents that augment dopamine, tolcapone increased dyskinesias, an effect noted most frequently during the first week of therapy but which gradually diminished in frequency and intensity as levodopa dosage was reduced. However, at 6 weeks, dyskinesia was still significantly more prevalent with tolcapone treatment compared to baseline and placebo. This increase may be explained in part by the relative

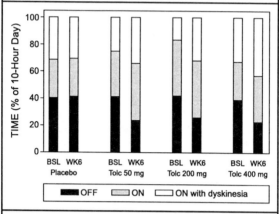

FIGURE 8.7 — MEAN "OFF" AND "ON" TIMES WITH AND WITHOUT DYSKINESIA: TOLCAPONE AND PLACEBO

Shown here are mean "off," "on," and "on with dyskinesia" times at baseline (BSL) and week 6 (WK6) as a percentage of the investigator-assessed 10-hour day. Patients were examined at 30-minute intervals for 10 hours (8 AM to 6 PM) at BSL and WK6. There was a statistically significant reduction in "off" time and an increase in both "on" and "on with dyskinesias" time for all three tolcapone doses, with no change in the placebo group.

Adapted from: Kurth MC, et al. *Neurology*. 1997;48:81-87.

brevity of the study, which limited reduction of levodopa dose.

All other side effects were dopaminergic in nature, including:

- Nausea
- Vomiting
- Postural hypotension
- Insomnia
- Confusion
- Hallucinations.

Most, if not all, can be expected to diminish as the levodopa regimen is adjusted.

Among 46 of these patients who participated in an arm of this study involving the evaluation of quality of life, all doses of tolcapone were associated with statistically significant improvement in total illness, physical illness, and psychosocial impact.[36]

Tolcapone as Early Therapy

Tolcapone has also been investigated as early therapy in patients on levodopa who have not yet experienced wearing-off phenomena.[37] The multicenter, double-blind, parallel-group, placebo-controlled study involved 298 patients who had been receiving levodopa plus carbidopa between 3 months and 5 years. The carbidopa/levodopa regimen had to have been stable for at least 4 weeks. All patients had shown clear improvement with the regimen and had UPDRS part II (activities of daily living) scores of 3 or more.

All patients received tolcapone, 100 mg or 200 mg, tid, for 6 months and at least 30% for 12 months. The primary efficacy variable was change in UPDRS part II, activities of daily living score. The sickness impact profile, change in daily levodopa dose, motor UPDRS, total UPDRS (I-III), and dyskinesias and fluctuations were secondary measures.

Both groups of tolcapone-treated patients showed significant reductions in UPDRS part II score compared with those on placebo. Total of UPDRS's parts I through III score, used as a measure of overall severity of impairment, was also significantly reduced in all treated patients, with the greatest improvement in the 200-mg group. The reduction in levodopa dose in tolcapone-treated patients began within the first 2 weeks of treatment and was maximal at 6 months. The development of motor fluctuations (assessed by proportion of day spent as "off" time) was seen in 11

8

119

(14%) of patients in the 200-mg group and 15 (19%) in the 100-mg group, compared to 20 (26%) in patients taking placebo.

In the 103 patients who completed 12 months of treatment, the reduction in levodopa dosage and improvements in UPDRS total and motor scores, as well as in activities of daily living seen at 6 months were maintained (Figure 8.8).

Most adverse events were mild or moderate. Fewer than 3% were severe, except for nausea in six patients and dyskinesia in one patient, all in the 200-mg group. Of 49 patients who withdrew from the study, 14 did so because of diarrhea: one from the placebo group and eight and five, respectively, from the 100-mg and 200-mg tolcapone groups. Diarrhea usually occurred 30 to 90 days after the initiation of treatment.

The only laboratory abnormality seen was raised liver enzymes (alanine aminotransferase) in three patients taking 100 mg of tolcapone, tid, and five taking 200 mg. Values returned to normal within 2 to 4 weeks in four patients who withdrew from the study on this account and resolved spontaneously in the four who continued treatment.

Dosage and Administration

Tolcapone should be given 100 or 200 mg, tid, q 6 hrs.

■ Entacapone (Comtan)

A peripherally acting COMT inhibitor, the experimental drug entacapone has been shown to increase the elimination half-life of levodopa and to increase "on" and decrease "off" times in patients with levodopa-related fluctuations. A number of both open label and randomized, double-blind studies have demonstrated that the drug:

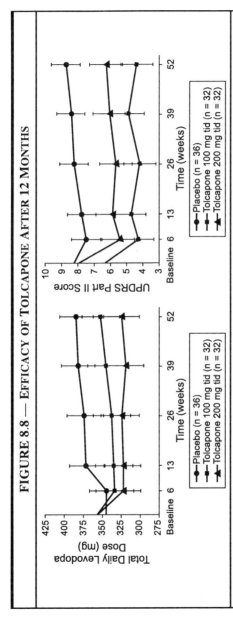

FIGURE 8.8 — EFFICACY OF TOLCAPONE AFTER 12 MONTHS

Both maximal reduction of levodopa dosage and improvements in activities of daily living achieved at 6 months were maintained at 12 months. Improvements in Unified Parkinson's Disease Rating Scale (UPDRS) total and motor scores were also maintained.

Adapted from: Waters CH, et al. *Neurology*. 1997;49:665-671.

8

- Prolongs the effect of levodopa
- Does not increase the magnitude of response to levodopa
- Does not delay patients' response to controlled-release (CR) carbidopa/levodopa.

In an open-label trial involving 15 parkinsonian patients with a fluctuating response to levodopa, chronic administration for 8 weeks resulted in reduction of the daily requirements for levodopa by 27%.[38] Patients reported a 77% daily "on" time, which dropped to 44% when the drug was withdrawn. Increased dyskinesia was common after introduction of entacapone but was managed by reducing levodopa.

In another, 4-week, open-label trial involving 12 patients with levodopa-related fluctuations, entacapone was shown to increase the duration of motor response to levodopa from 2.3 to 3.2 hours (39%) after a single dose and to 3.4 hours (48%) after 4 weeks.[39] The magnitude of clinical response remained unchanged, but peak latency of motor response was prolonged after 4 weeks. The duration and magnitude of dyskinesias also increased.

These results were validated in a 1-month crossover trial involving 23 patients given entacapone and placebo, each for 4 weeks.[40] Motor responses were repeatedly quantified using the motor part of UPDRS, and plasma levodopa and its metabolites were measured. Entacapone prolonged the availability of levodopa in the plasma and thus to the brain by decreasing peripheral O-methylation and slowing its elimination rate, without affecting the maximum plasma levodopa concentration or time to maximum concentration (Figure 8.9). Corresponding with the pharmacokinetic findings, entacapone drug prolonged the duration of a motor response to an individual dose of levodopa by 34 minutes (24%) and dyskinesias by 39 minutes (37%) compared with placebo, without

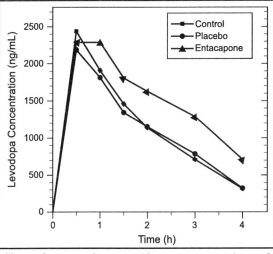

FIGURE 8.9 — PLASMA LEVODOPA CONCENTRATIONS DURING ADJUNCTIVE ENTACAPONE

Shown here are the mean plasma concentrations of levodopa after an individual oral dose of levodopa (with a levodopa decarboxylase inhibitor) alone (control day) and after 4 weeks of concomitant placebo or entacapone.

From: Ruottinen HM, Rinne UK. *J Neurol Neurosurg Psychiatry*. 1996;60:36-40.

affecting their magnitude or starting time. It resulted in a reduction of 16% in the mean total daily levodopa dose to minimize dyskinesias. Home diaries reported "on" time to be prolonged by 2.1 hours (Figure 8.10).

Finally, a randomized, double-blind, single-graded-dose, crossover trial of five 1-day treatment periods, each 1 week apart, of entacapone (50 mg, 100 mg, 200 mg, or 400 mg) and placebo was performed in 20 patients with levodopa-related fluctuations.[41] The inhibition of soluble COMT in red blood cells (RBCs) and plasma concentrations of levodopa,

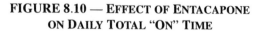

From: Ruottinen HM, Rinne UK. *J Neurol Neurosurg Psychiatry*. 1996;60:36-40.

FIGURE 8.10 — EFFECT OF ENTACAPONE ON DAILY TOTAL "ON" TIME

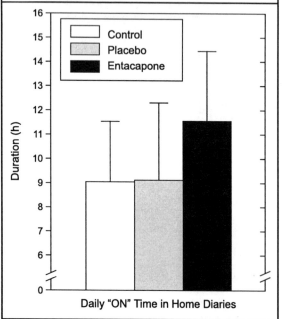

Mean "on" time reported in patients' home diaries was increased by approximately 2.1 hours among patients whose levodopa treatment regimen was supplemented by entacapone.

its metabolites, and entacapone were measured, and motor responses were quantified at 30-minute intervals using the motor part of the UPDRS. Results included:

- Entacapone was associated with a dose-dependent decrease in soluble COMT activity in RBCs, maximally by 48% at 400 mg.

- A 200-mg dose of entacapone resulted in increases in the area under the plasma concentration-time curve and half-life of levodopa (with decreases in the AUCs of 3-O-methyldopa and homovanillic acid and an increase in that of 3,4-dihydroxyphenylacetic acid.)
- Entacapone prolonged the duration of the motor response to levodopa by 33 minutes and dyskinesias by 45 minutes, without affecting their magnitude; the highest increase in duration was associated with the 200-mg dose.

Two large multicenter studies, conducted under the auspices of the Parkinson Study Group (North America) and the Nordic Study Group (Nordic countries), involved 205 and 171 patients, respectively, with motor fluctuations associated with levodopa therapy, particularly the "wearing-off" phenomenon, who received either entacapone, 200 mg, or placebo with each dose of levodopa for 24 weeks.[42,43] The primary measure of efficacy was a change in "on" time while awake, as recorded in patients' daily diaries at 30-minute intervals. Other outcome measures included change in UPDRS and clinical adverse effects. At baseline, patients averaged about 9 to 10 hours of "on" time (60.5% "on" time).

Results of the North American study included:
- Entacapone treatment increased the percent "on" time by 5.0 percentage points compared to placebo, nearly 1 extra hour a day, at weeks 8, 16, and 24.
- The effect of entacapone was more prominent in patients with a smaller baseline "on" time (< 55%).
- The effect of entacapone increased as the day wore on.

- At week 24, mean UPDRS scores were improved by approximately 10% among entacapone-treated patients compared to those on placebo.
- On withdrawal of entacapone, patients noted a complete and rapid loss of benefit.

Although transient dyskinesias and mild nausea were more common with entacapone treatment, this experimental drug was generally well tolerated, with no abnormalities in vital signs or laboratory surveillance tests. Entacapone was also effective in increasing the duration of response to levodopa.

Table 8.4 compares the COMT inhibitor agents.

TABLE 8.4 — COMT INHIBITORS		
	Entacapone	**Tolcapone**
COMT inhibition	Peripheral	Peripheral and central
Dosing	200 mg with every Levodopa dose	Fixed 100 mg to 200 mg tid
Elimination ($t_{\frac{1}{2}}$)	2 hours	2 hours
Adverse effects	• Nausea • Vomiting • Dyskinesias • Hypotension • Sedation • Headache • Constipation • Diarrhea	• Nausea • Vomiting • Dyskinesias • Sedation • Headache • Severe diarrhea occurring 6 to 8 weeks post initiation • Increased LFTs
Abbreviations: COMT, catechol-O-methyltransferase; LFT, liver function tests.		

Carbidopa/Levodopa

The immediate metabolic precursor of dopamine, levodopa (L-3,4-dihydroxyphenylalanine) is transported across the gut wall by a saturable, facilitated carrier system (the aromatic and branched chain "L" amino acid system).[6] More than 95% of levodopa is rapidly decarboxylated (an overall half-life of 1 hour) to dopamine in the periphery, however, so relatively little unchanged drug reaches the cerebral circulation and probably less than 1% actually crosses the blood-brain barrier to permeate into striatal tissue. Therefore, levodopa is almost always administered in combination with carbidopa, a peripheral inhibitor of dopa decarboxylase, to increase the fraction of unmetabolized drug available to cross the blood-brain barrier. This combination is called Sinemet.

Equally important, the addition of carbidopa has permitted an approximately 80% reduction in levodopa dosage, thus avoiding most of the nausea, vomiting, hypotension, sinus tachycardia, and orange urine that followed conversion of large doses to dopamine by the vascular endothelium.[2] The nausea and vomiting are mediated at the chemoreceptor trigger zone in the area postrema of the medulla, a region with no blood-brain barrier.

Despite levodopa's position as the gold standard for the symptomatic treatment of PD, the timing of its initiation remains somewhat controversial.[15] Theoretical reasons for delaying levodopa treatment include:

- The supposition that complications associated with levodopa are related to duration of treatment
- According to the oxidative stress hypothesis, levodopa may be feeding into the pathogenic mechanism by generating more dopamine and, in turn, more free radicals.

■ Duration of Treatment

Studies have reported differing results regarding the relationship between delaying levodopa treatment and the development of motor fluctuations or dyskinesias, including:[15]

- The rate of deterioration was the same whether levodopa was initiated early or late in the course of the disease.
- Dyskinesias occurred in a greater proportion of patients in whom the initiation of levodopa therapy was delayed by more than 2 years following diagnosis compared to those started earlier; furthermore, no adverse consequences of early treatment were found.
- In patients with severe MPTP-induced parkinsonism, dyskinesias and response fluctuations (see below) developed within the first few months of levodopa treatment, suggesting disease severity may be a determining factor.
- Prognosis was not adversely influenced by early levodopa treatment, and dyskinesias were related to severity of disease rather than early levodopa therapy.

■ Levodopa Toxicity

The concern regarding levodopa toxicity has led to recommendations that the drug be deferred until absolutely necessary and when it is finally instituted, that the lowest possible dose be given. Other clinicians have responded that such a strategy reduces patients' quality of life on the basis of an unproven theory.

The case against levodopa toxicity is contained in a number of study findings, including:[15]

- The longevity of PD patients increased with the introduction of levodopa therapy in the 1970s.

- Pathologic evidence of substantia nigra toxicity could not be detected in mice given large doses of levodopa for up to 18 months.
- When levodopa was administered for other conditions, there were no indications of its inducing irreversible clinical or pathologic deterioration.
- Pathologic changes in the substantia nigra of patients who had taken levodopa were no different from those of pre-levodopa patients.
- If dopamine, including that generated from levodopa therapy, is a major pathogenic source, why are the degenerative changes (and Lewy bodies) in brain regions that do not contain dopamine?
- With advancing disease, clinical deterioration often reflects cerebral degeneration in non-dopaminergic circuits (dementia, levodopa-refractory motor symptoms).
- If levodopa therapy hastens disease progression, the dopamine agonists, which do not generate dopamine, should result in less rapid disease progression than that associated with levodopa; however, similar rates of progression were found in a 1-year trial in which levodopa and the agonist bromocriptine were compared.
- Neither depletion nor megadose supplementation of the antioxidant tocopherol (vitamin E) has thus far been shown to have any significant influence on the development or progression of PD.

Thus, despite theoretical concerns, compelling evidence for levodopa toxicity has yet to be presented. Nevertheless, it seems judicious to respect this concern and to administer levodopa cautiously, without withholding it from patients in need. The treating physician's goal should be to keep patients within the mainstream of life if at all possible. Despite the on-going debate about when to begin levodopa, once the decision is made, there is little controversy regarding how the drug is to be introduced, titrated, and supplemented with adjunctive agents throughout the course of the disease.

Dosage and Administration

Carbidopa/levodopa treatment is usually started with

- One half of a 25/100 tablet, bid, after a meal
- Increased by ½ tablet/day every 4 to 7 days
- As dosage increases, 25/250 tablets can be substituted (only in rare cases are these large doses required). Initiating treatment with the higher dosage may cause:
  - Nausea
  - Dizziness
  - Insomnia
  - Nervousness
  - Vague mental symptoms.

Peripheral dopa decarboxylase is blocked by carbidopa at approximately 70 mg to 100 mg/day. Patients receiving less than that are likely to experience nausea and vomiting.

Realistically, treatment can usually abolish the disability caused by symptoms but cannot be expected to completely relieve symptoms. Therefore, patients must not be allowed to increase dosage on their own. Particularly in the later stages, in which long-term use of levodopa results in dyskinesia, they are likely to mistake the side effect for a worsening of disease and increase the dosage.

Side Effects

The most common serious adverse reactions occurring with carbidopa/levodopa are:

- Choreiform, dystonic, and other involuntary movements
- Mental changes, including paranoid ideation and psychotic episodes
- Nausea
- Cardiac irregularities
- Orthostatic hypotension
- Bradykinetic episodes (the "on-off" phenomena)
- Anorexia
- Vomiting
- Dizziness.

Controlled-Release Carbidopa/Levodopa

An estimated 10% of all patients treated with levodopa will develop motor fluctuations per year, resulting in 50% of patients being affected after 5 years of sustained therapy, many of whom may also experience drug-related involuntary movements as well.[44] These disorders may be related either to long-term levodopa therapy or to progression of the disease.

The mechanism(s) of motor response fluctuations, caused by both peripheral and central pharmacodynamic changes, are not completely understood, but variation in levodopa delivery appears to be a critical factor in their development. Continuous administration of levodopa has been shown to cause fewer behavioral changes and receptor alterations in both animal and clinical studies.

In a double-blind, 2-year study in untreated patients, a CR compound of levodopa and a dopa decarboxylase inhibitor was significantly better than an immediate-release (IR) preparation, with a lower occurrence of fluctuations and dyskinesia.[45] This finding was not confirmed, however, in another randomized, double-blind, multicenter study, which reported no differences in the occurrence of either motor fluctuations or dyskinesias in either treatment group followed for 5 years.

Finally, an international, 35-center, triple-blind, randomized, parallel comparison trial of IR and CR carbidopa/levodopa in 618 previously untreated PD patients has recently been reported.[43] The primary end point was progression of disease to the onset of motor fluctuations (the "event"), based on patient diaries and investigators' observations during quarterly clinic visits, noted on a standard motor fluctuation questionnaire (consisting of 10 questions related to "wearing-off" of drug effect). Other standardized methods of evaluating symptom severity, on a quarterly basis, were the:

- New York University Parkinson Disease Scale (NYUPDS)
- Northwestern University Disability Scale (NUDS)
- Hoehn and Yahr Stage and Schwab and England Activities of Daily Living Scale (annually)
- UPDRS (annually)
- Nottingham Health Profile (NHP, annually, in countries where validated translation exists).

Mean daily levodopa doses at baseline and after 5 years were:

- IR carbidopa/levodopa — 172 mg/day at baseline, 426 mg/day at 5 years
- CR carbidopa/levodopa — 345 mg/day (approximately 241 mg when corrected for bioavailability) at baseline and 728 mg/day at 5 years (approximately 510 when corrected for lower bioavailability of the preparation).

Investigators were allowed to make adjustments in the number and frequency of administration of tablets required to maintain an optimal clinical state. No significant differences in motor fluctuations were found between treatment groups, either by diary data or questionnaire. Other 5-year findings included:

- No clinically relevant changes between baseline and the 5-year evaluations on the NYUPDS, NUDS, and UPDRS.
- Approximately 30% of patients in each group maintained a twice-a-day dosing regimen; however, 25% of the IR patients required five or more doses a day compared to only 13% of the CR group.
- A statistically significant difference in activities of daily living as measured by the UPDRS in favor of CR carbidopa/levodopa.
- A statistically significant difference in favor of the CR preparation on NHP measures of emotional reaction and social isolation.
- No clinically relevant changes in global assessments (Hoehn-Yahr, Schwab-England scores) and no differences between treatment groups.
- Both groups showed statistically significant improvement over baseline during the early years, followed by slow erosion of performance to slightly worse than baseline around the end of the study.
- Overall incidence of withdrawal due to adverse events similar for two treatment groups (IR, 11%; CR, 8%); however no CR patients withdrew because of nausea, the most common side effect, compared to seven IR patients.

The investigators note that the CR preparation, because it provides a prolonged levodopa plasma concentration, should theoretically be associated with less motor fluctuations and dyskinesias. One explanation for their finding of few differences between the effects of the two preparations, as well as the conflicting results of previous studies lies in the existence of fluctuations that are independent of peak dose levodopa blood levels. Also, a difference between the two might be seen if a similar investigation were to be extended beyond 5 years.

Future Directions

An ethyl ester of levodopa has recently been shown to achieve higher striatal elevations and to last longer when injected subcutaneously into laboratory animals. It is suggested as a potential rescue strategy to overcome "off" situations in PD patients.[46]

Remacemide, the new nondopaminergic glutamate receptor antagonist, an anticonvulsant, neuroprotective compound, has been shown to ameliorate motor symptoms of MPTP-induced parkinsonism in animal models.

Current concepts of basal ganglia circuitry predict that degeneration of nigrostriatal neurons disinhibits downstream sites like the subthalamic nucleus (STN).[47] The ability of subthalamic lesions to decrease tremor, rigidity, and akinesia in the contralateral limbs of monkeys with MPTP-induced parkinsonism supports this notion and suggests overactivity of the STN may be responsible for symptoms in PD. And subthalamic overactivity involves an increase in glutamate-mediated neurotransmission; antagonists of NMDA/glutamate receptors have been shown to enhance the ability of levodopa to reverse akinesia and rigidity in rats treated with catecholamine-depleting agents, such as reserpine. (Studies using a variety of glutamate-receptor subtype-selective agonists and antagonists implicated both NMDA and non-NMDA receptors located at different sites in the basal ganglia.)

Remacemide potentiates the antiparkinsonian effects of carbidopa/levodopa in reserpinized rats and MPTP-treated monkeys by blocking NMDA/glutamate receptors in the STN. In contrast to some other NMDA antagonists, remacemide does not produce lo-

134

comotor stimulation in normal rats, possibly because its affinity for NMDA channels is lower than that of classic blockers. Thus, it dissociates rapidly from NMDA channels, potentially reducing the severity or duration of psychotomimetic and other adverse drug effects.

Remacemide had no antiparkinsonian effects when administered alone to monoamine-depleted rats.[48] When combined with a subthreshold dose of levodopa methyl ester, however, it increased motor activity dramatically in dose-dependent fashion. Furthermore, low doses of remacemide were shown to reduce the requirement for dopaminergic therapy in rodent and primate models of PD.

The drug's possibly neuroprotective effect is based on the "excitotoxic" theory, which states that a defect in mitochondrial energy metabolism could secondarily lead to slow excitotoxic neuronal death by making neurons more vulnerable to endogenous glutamate (see Chapter 6, *Pathophysiology*).[49]

Remacemide has good oral bioavailability and is well tolerated in humans. The Parkinson Study Group, a consortium of university-based movement disorder centers in the United States and Canada, is currently sponsoring a multicenter safety and efficacy study of remacemide in the treatment of PD.

REFERENCES

1. Koller WC. Treatment of Parkinson's disease: mild and moderate treatment options. Syllabus, Course 127. American Academy of Neurology Annual Meeting; 1995; Seattle, Wash.

2. Golbe LI, Sage JI. Medical treatment of Parkinson's disease. In: Kurlan R, ed. *Treatment of Movement Disorders*. Philadelphia, Pa: JB Lippencott Co; 1995:1-56.

3. Hurtig HI. Problems with current pharmacologic treatment of Parkinson's disease. *Exp Neurol*. 1997;144:10-16.

4. Calne DB. Initiating treatment for idiopathic parkinsonism. *Neurology*. 1994;44(7 suppl 6):S19-S22.

5. Stern MB. Contemporary approaches to the pharmacotherapeutic management of Parkinson's disease: an overview. *Neurology*. 1997;49(1 suppl 1):S2-S9.

6. Standaert DG, Young AB. Treatment of central nervous system degenerative disorders: Parkinson's disease. In: Hardman JG, Limbird LE, Molinoff NB, Ruddon RW, Gilmon AG, eds. *Goodman and Gilman's The Pharmacological Basis of Therapeutics*. 9th ed. New York, NY: McGraw-Hill; 1996:506-513.

7. Blanpied TA, Boeckman FA, Aizenman E, Johnson JW. Trapping channel block of NMDA-activated responses by amantadine and memantine. *J Neurophysiol*. 1997;77:309-323.

8. The Parkinson Study Group. Effect of deprenyl on the progression of disability in early Parkinson's disease. *N Engl J Med*. 1989;321:1364-1371.

9. Parkinson Study Group. Impact of deprenyl and tocopherol treatment on Parkinson's disease in DATATOP patients requiring levodopa. *Ann Neurol*. 1996;39:37-45.

10. Koller WC. Neuroprotective therapy for Parkinson's disease. *Exp Neurol*. 1997;144:24-28.

11. Olanow CW. Attempts to obtain neuroprotection in Parkinson's disease. *Neurology*. 1997;49(1 suppl 1):S26-S33.

12. Tatton WG, Wadia JS, Ju WY, Chalmers-Redman RM, Tatton NA. (-)-Deprenyl reduces neuronal apoptosis and facilitates neuronal outgrowth by altering protein synthesis without inhibiting monoamine oxidase. *J Neural Transm*. 1996;48 (suppl):45-59.

13. Wu RM, Murphy DL, Chiueh CC. Suppression of hydroxyl radical formation and protection of nigral neurons by 1-deprenyl (selegiline). *Ann N Y Acad Sci*. 1996;786:379-390.

14. Le W, Jankovic J. Xie W, Kong R, Appel SH. (-)-Deprenyl protection of 1-methyl-4 phenylpyridium ion (MPP+)-induced apoptosis independent of MAO-B inhibition. *Neurosci Lett*. 1997;224:197-200.

15. Ahlskog JE. Treatment options for mild and moderate Parkinson's disease. Syllabus, Course 236. American Academy of Neurology 48th Annual Meeting; San Francisco, Calif; 1996:25-42.

16. Lees AJ. Comparison of therapeutic effects and mortality data of levodopa and levodopa combined with selegiline in patients with early, mild Parkinson's disease. Parkinson's Disease Research Group of the United Kingdom. *BMJ*. 1995;311: 1602-1607.

17. de Rijk MC, Breteler MM, den Breeijen JH, et al. Dietary antioxidants and Parkinson disease. The Rotterdam Study. *Arch Neurol*. 1997;54:762-765.

18. Mizuno Y, Kondo T, Narabayashi H. Pergolide in the treatment of Parkinson's disease. *Neurology*. 1995;45(3 suppl 3):S13-S21.

19. Mierau J, Schneider FJ, Ensinger HA, Chio CL, Lajiness ME, Huff RM. Pramipexole binding and activation of cloned and expressed dopamine D_2, D_3 and D_4 receptors. *Eur J Pharmacol*. 1995;290:29-36.

20. Hubble JP, Koller WC, Cutler NR, et al. Pramipexole in patients with early Parkinson's disease. *Clin Neuropharmacol*. 1995;18:338-347.

21. Shannon KM, Bennett JP Jr, Friedman JH. Efficacy of pramipexole, a novel dopamine agonist, as monotherapy in mild to moderate Parkinson's disease. The Pramipexole Study Group. *Neurology*. 1997;49:724-728.

22. Parkinson Study Group. Safety and efficacy of pramipexole in early Parkinson disease. A randomized dose-ranging study. *JAMA*. 1997;278:125-130.

23. Molho ES, Factor SA, Weiner WJ, et al. The use of pramipexole, a novel dopamine (DA) agonist, in advanced Parkinson's disease. *J Neural Transm*. 1995;45(suppl):225-230.

24. Lieberman A, Ranhosky A, Korts D. Clinical evaluation of pramipexole in advanced Parkinson's disease: results of a double-blind, placebo-controlled, parallel-group study. *Neurology*. 1997;49:162-168.

25. Guttman M. Double-blind comparison of pramipexole and bromocriptine treatment with placebo in advanced Parkinson's disease. *Neurology.* 1997;49:1060-1065.

26. Tulloch IF. Pharmacologic profile of ropinirole: a nonergoline dopamine agonist. *Neurology.* 1997;49(1 suppl 1):S58-S62.

27. Rascol O. Ropinirole: clinical profile. In: Olanow CW, Obeso JA, eds. *Beyond the Decade of the Brain.* Vol 2. Royal Tunbridge Wells, UK: Wells Medical Limited; 1997:163-175.

28. Adler CH, Sethi KD, Hauser RA, et al. Ropinirole for the treatment of early Parkinson's disease. The Ropinirole Study Group. *Neurology.* 1997;49: 393-399.

29. Rascol O. A double-blind, L-dopa-controlled study of ropinirole in patients with early Parkinson's disease. *Neurology.* 1996;46:A160. Abstract.

30. Korczyn AD. A double-blind study comparing ropinirole and bromocriptine in patients with early Parkinson's disease. *Neurology.* 1996;46:A159. Abstract.

31. Korczyn AD, Brooks DJ, Brunt ER. Ropinirole vs. bromocriptine in the early treatment of Parkinson's disease: a six-month interim report of a three-year study. *Mov Disord.* 1998; 13:in press.

32. Rascol O, Brooks DJ, Brunt ER. Ropinirole in the early treatment of Parkinson's disease: a six-month interim report on a five-year L-dopa controlled study. *Mov Disord.* 1998;13:in press.

33. Kreider MS, Willson-Lynch K, Gardiner D, Wheadon DE. A double-blind, placebo-controlled extension study to evaluate the 12-month efficacy and safety of ropinirole in early Parkinson's disease. *Neurology.* 1997;48:A269. Abstract.

34. Rascol O, Lees AJ, Senard JM, Pirtosek Z, Montastruc JL, Fuell D. Ropinirole in the treatment of levodopa-induced motor fluctuations in patients with Parkinson's disease. *Clin Neuropharmacol.* 1996;19:234-245.

35. Kurth MC, Adler CH, Hilaire MS, et al. Tolcapone improves motor function and reduces levodopa requirement in patients with Parkinson's disease experiencing motor fluctuations: a multicenter, double-blind, randomized, placebo-controlled trial. Tolcapone Fluctuator Study Group I. *Neurology.* 1997;48:81-87.

36. Welsh MD, Ved N, Waters CH. Psychosocial adjustment and illness impact in Parkinson's disease patients before and after treatment with tolcapone (Tasmar). *Neurology.* 1996;46: A322. Abstract.

37. Waters CH, Kurth M, Bailey P, et al. Tolcapone in stable Parkinson's disease: efficacy and safety of long-term treatment. *Neurology.* 1997;49:665-671.

38. Nutt JG, Woodward WR, Beckner RM, et al. Effect of peripheral catechol-O-methyltransferase inhibition on the pharmacokinetics and pharmacodynamics of levodopa in parkinsonian patients. *Neurology.* 1994;44:913-919.

39. Ruottinen HM, Rinne UK. Effect of one month's treatment with peripherally acting catechol-O-methyltransferase inhibitor, entacapone, on pharmacokinetics and motor response to levodopa in advanced parkinsonian patients. *Clin Neuropharmacol.* 1996;19:222-233.

40. Ruottinen HM, Rinne UK. Entacapone prolongs levodopa response in a one month double blind study in parkinsonian patients with levodopa related fluctuations. *J Neurol Neurosurg Psychiatry.* 1996;60:36-40.

41. Ruottinen HM, Rinne UK. A double-blind pharmacokinetic and clinical dose-response study of entacapone as an adjuvant to levodopa therapy in advanced Parkinson's disease. *Clin Neuropharmacol.* 1996;19:283-296.

42. Kieburtz K (Parkinson Study Group), Rinne UK (Nordic Study Group). The COMT-inhibitor entacapone increases "on" time in levodopa-treated PD patients with motor fluctuations: report of two randomized, placebo-controlled trials. *Mov Disord.* 1996;11:595-596.

43. Parkinson Study Group. The COMT inhibitor entacapone improves motor fluctuations in patients with levodopa-treated Parkinson's disease. *Ann Neurol.* 1997;42:747-755.

44. Block G, Liss C, Reines S, Irr J, Nibbelink D. Comparison of immediate-release and controlled release carbidopa/levodopa in Parkinson's disease. A multicenter 5-year study. The CR First Study Group. *Eur Neurol*. 1997;37:23-27.

45. Djaldetti R, Atlas D, Melamed E. Effect of subcutaneous administration of levodopa ethyl ester, a soluble prodrug of levodopa, on dopamine metabolism in rodent striatum: implication for treatment of Parkinson's disease. *Clin Neuropharmacol*. 1996;19:65-71.

46. Greenberg DA. Glutamate and Parkinson's disease. *Ann Neurol*. 1994;35:639. Editorial.

47. Greenamyre JT, Eller RV, Zhang Z, Oradia A, Kurlan R, Gash DM. Antiparkinsonian effects of remacemide hydrochloride, a glutamate antagonist, in rodent and primate models of Parkinson's disease. *Ann Neurol*. 1994;35:655-661.

48. Beal MF. Does impairment of energy metabolism result in excitotoxic neuronal death in neurodegenerative illnesses? *Ann Neurol*. 1992;31:119-130.

9 Complications of Parkinson's Disease and Its Therapy

Consideration of the essentially inevitable treatment-related motor complications of later-stage Parkinson's disease (PD) shapes primary therapeutic interventions and is very much part of everyday management. A host of other side effects — behavioral, hypotensive, and gastrointestinal — which may have no affect on motor function, can significantly alter that treatment plan. Both motor and nonmotor complications will be summarized here.

Levodopa Dose-Related Motor Fluctuations

During the early years of levodopa treatment, patients should be questioned routinely about signs of "wearing-off" response or dyskinesias.[1] Specifically, each patient should be asked about return of minimal tremor, bradykinesia, voice softness, or decreased manual dexterity after a dose of levodopa. The first sign of beginning fluctuations may be heralded by:

- Early morning akinesia
- Loss of sleep benefit (the refreshing effects of sleep)
- Restlessness or fidgetiness (early signs of peak-dose chorea)
- Internal tremor as an end-of-dose pattern.

Motor abnormalities are influenced by peripheral and central levodopa pharmacokinetics and central pharmacodynamic influences (Table 9.1).[2] Gas-

TABLE 9.1 — POSSIBLE MECHANISMS OF LEVODOPA-RELATED MOTOR FLUCTUATIONS

- Peripheral pharmacokinetic
  - Delayed gastric emptying
  - Protein competition
- Central pharmacokinetic
  - Variations in striatal levodopa levels (reduced storage)
  - Damage to dopaminergic neurons by toxic by-products of dopamine metabolism
- Central pharmacodynamic
  - Altered dopamine receptors
  - Altered dopamine-receptor sensitivity profile

Adapted from: Waters CH. *Neurology*. 1997;49(1 suppl 1):S49-S57.

trointestinal activity is crucial to the delivery of levodopa to the brain.[1] Since absorption of levodopa occurs mostly in the duodenum and jejunum, erratic gastric emptying is a controlling factor. Under certain conditions, it may result in lower plasma levodopa concentrations or may be responsible for some biphasic absorption patterns. Factors that affect gastric emptying are:

- Increased gastric acidity
- Antiparkinsonian drugs (primarily anticholinergics)
- Food.

Levodopa is transported from gut to blood and across the blood-brain barrier on the large, neutral amino acid carrier system. With normal food intake, concentrations of neutral amino acids in blood are near saturation for blood-brain transport. Therefore, food-derived amino acids have the potential to interfere with levodopa transport. For example:

- Protein loads with significant amounts of neutral amino acids can interfere with levodopa uptake.
- Physical activity may reduce mesenteric blood flow, decreasing levodopa absorption and worsening fluctuations.

Factors affecting central pharmacokinetics include pulsatile delivery of levodopa to striatal receptors and impaired storage capacity of dopamine, caused by the progressive loss of nigral neurons. During the first few years of levodopa therapy, symptoms tend to improve and remain under stable control on infrequent dosing, 2 or 3 times a day. The remaining nigrostriatal neurons provide adequate dopamine storage capacity, and the brain retains its ability to buffer swings in cerebral levodopa availability. Within 3 to 5 years, however, with increased nigral cell death, levodopa's efficacy begins to decline (Figure 9.1).[3] There is a gradual but unpredictable tendency for the early, smooth response to levodopa to give way to the nonphysiologic, short-duration response, which emerges as a subtle — later, a more pronounced — pattern of "wearing off" and "on/off" motor fluctuations complicated by abnormal involuntary movements or dyskinesias (Figure 9.2).[4] More frequent or larger doses of levodopa result in striatal receptor supersensitivity and an altered balance between dopamine receptor subtypes.[2]

It has been suggested that reduced dopamine storage is contributory to but not directly responsible for the fluctuating response to levodopa.[5] Although the minimal effective dose of the drug appears not to change overtime or with increasing severity of disease, the dyskinesia threshold is lowered. Moreover, the threshold is much lower in patients who experience fluctuations than in those who remain stable. Thus, the drug seems to create its antiparkinsonian effect and

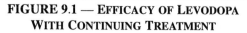

FIGURE 9.1 — EFFICACY OF LEVODOPA WITH CONTINUING TREATMENT

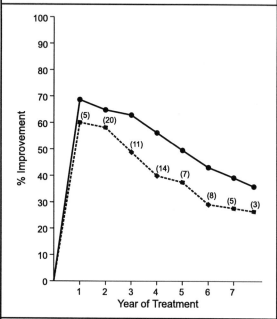

In a retrospective study of 597 patients on long-term levodopa therapy, Parkinson signs improved dramatically in the first year, were sustained for about 3 years, then began to decline (solid line). The course of the 73 patients who died (dotted line) is compared with the total group. Number who died each year is noted in parentheses.

Adapted from: Fahn S. In: Rowland LP, ed. *Merritt's Textbook of Neurology*. 1995:713-730.

to produce dyskinesias through separate mechanisms, probably via different dopamine receptor subtypes. D_1 (excitatory) receptors are associated with dyskinesias, whereas stimulation of D_2 (inhibitory) receptors by the D_2 dopamine agonists results in motor benefits with less dyskinesia than occurs with levodopa.[6] The motor abnormalities include:[2]

144

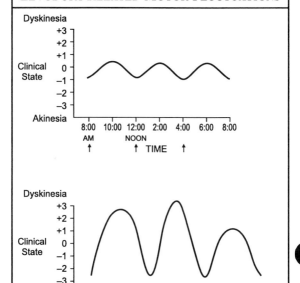

FIGURE 9.2 — DEVELOPMENT OF LEVODOPA-RELATED MOTOR FLUCTUATIONS

After 3 to 5 years of treatment with levodopa, it is associated with mild "on-off" motor fluctuations (top). As the disease progresses and levodopa treatment continues, the fluctuations increase dramatically, with prominent swings between severe akinesia and pronounced dyskinesia (bottom). Arrows indicate dosing times.

Adapted from: Hurtig HI. *Exp Neurol.* 1997;144:10-16.

- "Wearing-off" fluctuations
- "On-off" fluctuations
- Dyskinesias
- Drug-failure response
- Beginning-of-dose deterioration
- Freezing
- Falls.

Management strategies for some of these motor complications are listed in Table 9.2.[2]

TABLE 9.2 — TREATMENT OF MOTOR COMPLICATIONS OF PARKINSON'S DISEASE

Motor Response	Management
"Wearing-off"	• More frequent dosing of levodopa • COMT inhibitor • Dopamine agonist • Controlled-release levodopa
"Off"-period dystonia	• Controlled-release levodopa • Dopamine agonist • COMT inhibitor • Dietary adjustments
"On-off"	• Liquid levodopa • Dopamine agonist • Clozapine
Drug failure	• Domperidone (where available) • Cisapride
Peak-dose dyskinesia/ dystonia	• Reduce each dose of levodopa • Use dopamine agonist • Add anticholinergic
Abbreviations: COMT, catechol-O-methyltransferase.	
Adapted from: Waters CH. *Neurology*. 1997;49(1 suppl 1):S49-S57.	

■ **"Wearing-Off" Fluctuations**

The "wearing-off" phenomenon, an increasingly shortened benefit period following each dose of levodopa, is the most common type of motor fluctuation seen in PD patients. Linked to nigrostriatal system degeneration, it is regular and predictable and occurs 2 to 4 hours after a levodopa dose (Figure 9.3). The effective time for the antiparkinsonian effects of levodopa correlates inversely with the overall sever-

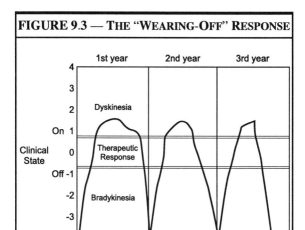

FIGURE 9.3 — THE "WEARING-OFF" RESPONSE

The typical wearing-off response, an increasingly short-ened benefit period following each dose of levodopa is the most common motor fluctuation. The length of be-tween-dose efficacy correlates inversely with the overall severity of parkinsonian signs, a presumptive index of the degree of nigrostriatal dopamine system loss.

Adapted from: Waters CH. *Neurology.* 1997;49(1 suppl 1):S49-S57.

ity of parkinsonian signs, a presumptive index of the degree of nigrostriatal dopamine system loss.

Patients experiencing the "wearing-off" period may present with sensory, psychiatric, and autonomic as well as motor fluctuations (Figure 9.4). Paresthe-sia, pain, tachycardia, sweating, constipation, belch-ing, and shortness of breath commonly occur during "off" periods and, if not recognized as part of the levodopa response pattern, may result in the ordering of unnecessary diagnostic tests. For example, many patients who complain of shortness of breath undergo extensive pulmonary evaluations only to discover that this symptom is actually caused by levodopa's "wear-

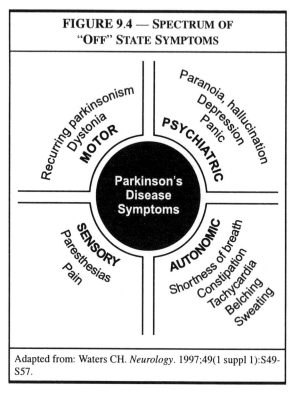

FIGURE 9.4 — SPECTRUM OF "OFF" STATE SYMPTOMS

Recurring parkinsonism
Dystonia
MOTOR

Paranoia, hallucination
Depression
Panic
PSYCHIATRIC

Parkinson's Disease Symptoms

SENSORY
Paresthesias
Pain

AUTONOMIC
Shortness of breath
Constipation
Tachycardia
Belching
Sweating

Adapted from: Waters CH. *Neurology.* 1997;49(1 suppl 1):S49-S57.

ing-off" phenomenon. A patient log of dosage schedules and symptoms would have revealed the same information less expensively and less invasively.

Management

Strategies for managing "wearing-off" phenomena focus on adjusting the medication dose for optimal effect. Patients with short-duration responses often respond well to the adjunctive therapy with a dopamine agonist. Dopamine agonists improve antiparkinsonian efficacy and smooth out fluctuations in response by directly stimulating postsynaptic dopamine receptors. Motor problems often can be improved by adjusting the ratio of the dose of levodopa to that of the dopamine agonist, depending on which is better tolerated.

Lowering individual doses of levodopa and shortening the dosage interval so that the total daily dosage remains unchanged works well initially; unfortunately, with time, the dosage interval may become inconveniently short. Prolonged-release levodopa preparations may be substituted in part or totally for the immediate-release levodopa previously used. However, when switching from regular to controlled-release (CR) preparations, the levodopa dosage must be increased. Reduced bioavailability requires a daily levodopa dose of about $1^1/_3$ times that of immediate release levodopa for most patients.

Patients who do well for most of the day on CR carbidopa/levodopa but have trouble with early-morning akinesia may benefit from taking the immediate-release preparation along with the CR dose first thing in the morning. This regimen "jump starts" the day for these patients, preparing them physically for normal activities.

Catechol-O-methyltransferase (COMT) inhibitors are also useful for wearing-off phenomena. Selegiline can be considered here.

When motor fluctuations are severe, transition to liquid carbidopa may be considered (see *Management* of *On-Off Fluctuations*). Finally, adding amantadine may mildly improve short-duration responses.

■ **On-Off Fluctuations**

"On-off" fluctuations are characterized by sudden, unpredictable shifts between undertreated and overtreated states. These motor shifts may be an indirect result of the alteration of presynaptic dopamine terminals resulting from fluctuating transmitter levels.

Management

Because they are sudden and unpredictable, "on-off" responses are difficult to treat. The addition or increased dosage of a dopamine agonist or larger doses of levodopa can be tried; however, most pharmacologic interventions that improve the "on" time will increase dyskinesias. An exception is clozapine, which may reduce dyskinesias in advanced PD.

Changing to liquid levodopa can be considered in patients with severe fluctuations that cannot be managed with the above measures. Liquid levodopa may allow more consistent and reliable control.[7] Close titration is possible with this strategy and may result in less "off" time and potentially fewer dyskinesias. This option, though, is viable only in highly motivated patients who are willing to accept the inconvenience of very frequent dosing and daily preparation. Because commercial products are unavailable, the solution must be prepared daily:

- Pulverize ten 25/100 mg standard-release carbidopa/levodopa tablets and 2 g of ascorbic acid.
- Combine the powder with 1 liter of tap water.
- Administer in small doses at 60- to 90-minute intervals, titrated to response; total daily dose should equal that prescribed in tablet formulation.

■ Dyskinesias

Dyskinesias are drug- and disease-related. Exclusively dystonic movements in the absence of chorea are common in PD and can be caused by the disease process itself or, frequently, by undertreated parkinsonism. Choreiform/choreodystonic dyskinesias invariably are related to long-term levodopa therapy. Dyskinesia usually occurs at the peak-dose concentration of levodopa, although sometimes it presents during the intervals between "off" and "on" responses.

Like the "wearing-off" phenomenon, dyskinesia indicates changes in striatal bioavailability of levodopa, signified by a rough correlation between plasma levels of levodopa and symptom presentation. Patterns of dyskinesia can be detected by observing patients for several days. Levodopa-induced dyskinesias may be classified into three main categories:

- "On" dyskinesias, characterized by chorea, myoclonus, and dystonic movements
- Diphasic dyskinesias, stereotyped, repetitive movements of the lower limbs
- "Off" dyskinesias, characterized by dystonic postures, especially of the feet.

Diphasic dyskinesia (dyskinesia-improvement-dyskinesia syndrome) is a variation in which patients experience dyskinesias at the beginning as well as at the end of an interval following the levodopa dose, corresponding to levodopa levels as they rise and fall. In one study that assessed levodopa-related dyskinesias in 168 patients, those associated with repetitive, alternating movements were exclusively associated with diphasic dyskinesia; dystonic postures of the limbs occurred only in "off" states, and chorea was the predominant feature of "on" states (Table 9.3).[8]

"Off" dystonia, especially lower limb dystonia, often is most troublesome when patients wake in the morning. They may develop twisting dystonic movements in one leg during the day, increasing their chances of stumbling. Lower-limb dystonia usually resolves after the first daily dose of levodopa.

Management

The first approach to treating dyskinesias is to modestly lower individual doses of levodopa (in 25 mg increments). Addition of a dopamine agonist may

TABLE 9.3 — PRESENTATION PATTERNS OF LEVODOPA-RELATED DYSKINESIAS AMONG 168 PATIENTS

Type	Presentation		
	"On"	Diphasic	"Off"
Chorea	113	0	0
Dystonic movements (limbs)	18	0	0
Craniocervical dystonia	13	0	2
Blepharospasm	4	1	1
Mixed movement disorders	9	0	0
Myoclonus	6	0	0
Tics	1	0	0
Repetitive alternating movements	0	24	0
Dystonic postures (limbs)	0	6	57

Adapted from: Luquin MR, et al. *Mov Disord*. 1992;7:117-124.

allow for reduced levodopa dosage without compromising symptomatic control. Diphasic dyskinesias may require a liquid levodopa regimen.

■ Drug Failure

Drug failure response to levodopa is a phenomenon that occurs in the late afternoon and may be related to poor gastric emptying and inadequate absorption. Treatment options include domperidone, where available, and cisapride, which augments gastric motility.

■ Beginning-of-Dose Deterioration

Patients may report a 20-minute or so worsening of symptoms after taking levodopa. This seems to be a transient effect that does not require treatment.[9]

■ Freezing

Considered to be a type of akinesia, freezing takes many forms. Patients may have difficulty with starting to walk (start hesitation); they may suddenly "freeze" in doorways, while crossing the street, and on turning. The problem may occur at any time, is worsened by stress, and may result in falls.

Freezing may occur during either "on" or "off" states. "On" freezing is poorly understood, and although "off" freezing is a manifestation of PD, unlike the other characteristic signs, it does not respond readily to levodopa. That freezing may reflect a deficiency in another neurotransmitter, norepinephrine, has been suggested, but treatment of the deficiency with a norepinephrine precursor has been unsatisfactory.

Other suggestions to overcome freezing include auditory, visual (parallel lines on the walking surface), and proprioceptive cues. In one study, an inverted walking stick helped some patients.

■ Falls

Postural instability is one of the cardinal features of relatively advanced PD. This symptom does not respond to levodopa, which, to the contrary, may actually contribute to the problem by allowing patients sufficient mobility to ambulate.

■ Other Motor Abnormalities

A recent review article outlined six phenomena related to motor fluctuations that had not been described previously.[10]

- Severe burning pain (like a fresh sunburn), which was misdiagnosed as fibrositis and was relieved by carbidopa/levodopa
- Restless legs, accompanied by kicking and shaking, which occurred at regular intervals at the end of each carbidopa/levodopa dose;

153

symptoms resolved with a change to the CR form

- Severe urinary urgency and frequency when carbidopa/levodopa wore off, accompanied by slowness and gait difficulties
- Depression, crying spells, and restlessness when the medication wore off
- Development of an anxiety state similar to a panic attack (tension, nervousness, chest pressure, breathing difficulty); this patient also had urinary complaints and cyclical suicidal thoughts; symptoms improved with medication adjustments
- Moaning and screaming accompanied by anxiety and confusion, all of which improved with a change to the CR preparation.

Behavioral/Psychiatric Disorders

The major neuropsychiatric disorders associated with advanced PD include:[2]

- Dementia
- Depression
- Hallucinations
- Psychoses
- Sleep disturbances.

The neuropsychiatric manifestations of PD can be more disabling than the motor dysfunctions. Before deciding on a management approach to an individual patient, it is necessary to ascertain whether the symptoms are induced by medication (hallucinations), related to disease state (depression, "off" state anxiety), or a combination of disease state and exacerbation by medication (memory loss, confusion). The presumptive cause will dictate whether or not the addition of a psychoactive medication is warranted or if reduction in dosage of one or more antiparkinsonian agents is needed (Table 9.4).

■ **Dementia**

The dementia associated with PD has been estimated to affect at least 20% of patients, with prevalence higher among older patients, rare among those with young-onset disease. Although distinctions are

TABLE 9.4 — TREATMENT OF BEHAVIORAL/PSYCHIATRIC DISORDERS ASSOCIATED WITH PARKINSON'S DISEASE

Behavioral/ Psychiatric Disorder	Management
Depression	• Antidepressant — Use: – Stimulating antidepressant if apathy is major feature – Sedating antidepressant if sleep disturbance is major feature
Hallucinations and psychosis	• Reduce or stop: – Adjunctive medications (eg, amantadine, anticholinergics) – Dopamine agonist • Reduce dosage of levodopa • Clozapine • Olanzapine
Sleep Disorders	
Sleep fragmentation	• Controlled-release carbidopa/levodopa • Sedating antidepressant • Benzodiazepine
Nocturnal vocalizations/vivid dreams	• Reduce dopaminergic medications near bedtime
Daytime sleepiness	• Increase activity • Caffeine

Adapted from: Waters CH. *Neurology.* 1997;49(1 suppl 1):S49-S57.

9

often blurred, Parkinson's dementia should be clinically distinguishable from that of Alzheimer's disease.[9] The *cortical* dementia of Alzheimer's is characterized by:

- Memory loss
- Aphasia
- Apraxia
- Agnosia.

The *subcortical* dementia is differentiated by a syndrome of:

- Poor concentration and initiative
- Memory loss (a confusing similarity)
- Slow responses (bradyphemia).

Functional imaging with single photon emission computed tomography (SPECT) or positron emission tomography (PET) is rarely helpful in clarifying the diagnosis since results are similar in all types of dementia.

Dementia is associated with a poorer prognosis for survival in Parkinson's patients. These patients respond poorly to levodopa and experience frequent side effects, and their disability progresses rapidly.

In the differential diagnosis of a parkinsonian patient with dementia, diffuse Lewy body disease must also be considered (see Chapter 7, *Diagnosis*).

Before treating PD-related dementia, it is crucial to eliminate all reversible causes of dementia, such as:

- Vitamin B_{12} deficiency
- Hypothyroidism
- Neurosyphilis
- Normal pressure hydrocephalus
- Mass lesions.

Thus, a routine dementia workup is warranted. All medications should be reassessed, and all antiparkinsonian medications should be eliminated except for carbidopa/levodopa, at the lowest possible dosage.

The anticholinergic agents must be avoided and should be eliminated in anyone complaining of memory loss. The new cholinesterase inhibitor, donepezil (Aricept), has not been tested in the dementia associated with PD.

■ **Depression**

An estimated 40% to 60% of patients suffer from depression, which appears to be related to duration of disease. Whether depression is related to the loss of frontal dopaminergic projections or serotonin deficiency or is a psychological response to PD has not yet been resolved.[2] However, depression is clearly related to the "off" periods of levodopa response and lifts with improved control of motor symptoms. Before prescribing any antidepressant, it is important to consider any possible drug interactions with patients' antiparkinson medication.

Patients with PD and depression usually respond to treatment with conventional antidepressants. Sedating agents (the tricyclics) are useful for patients with sleep disorders, whereas those with apathetic depression may be helped by a more stimulating selective serotonin uptake inhibitor (SSRI).

Anticholinergic and orthostatic adverse effects may limit the effectiveness or prevent the use of tricyclic agents (TCAs) in elderly patients. Of the available TCAs, trazodone has a lower anticholinergic potential and is often the better choice for these patients.

The four available SSRIs are:
- Fluoxetine (Prozac)
- Sertraline (Zoloft)
- Paroxetine (Paxil)
- Venlafaxine (Effexor).

Two other SSRIs, nefazodone (Serzone) and fluvoxamine (Luvox) are also available, but little information regarding their use in PD patients has been reported. Amoxapine (Asendin) should be avoided because of a potential as a dopamine receptor blocker, it has produced neuroleptic malignant syndrome in patients with PD.[11,12]

Finally, because there is a potential for a drug-drug interaction between SSRIs and selegiline, concurrent use is discouraged.[2]

Troublesome side effects of fluoxetine include:
- Nervousness
- Anxiety
- Dizziness.

Although there are rare reports of fluoxetine's worsening PD, albeit reversibly with discontinuation of the drug, a recent prospective study showed no aggravation of symptoms or signs among 14 patients treated with 20 mg/day.[13] No information is available concerning the use of sertraline in patients with PD, and one recent report associates paroxetine with aggravating parkinsonism.

At least two studies have reported the successful use of electroconvulsive therapy (ECT) in severely depressed Parkinson patients.[14,15] Whether this is a true phenomenon is not yet clear given the confounding variable in the studies. However, ECT may be the treatment of choice for severely depressed patients who have failed medical management or who have intolerable side effects or confusion in response to an antidepressant.

■ Hallucinations and Psychosis
Psychiatric adverse effects are much more likely to occur in patients with predisposing characteristics such as:

- Dementia
- Advanced age
- Premorbid psychiatric illness
- Exposure to high daily doses of levodopa.[2]

Excessive levodopa may cause hallucinations or psychosis in all patients with PD. Other antiparkinsonian drugs have been implicated in various forms of psychosis, including:
- Bromocriptine
- Pergolide
- Apomorphine
- Pramipexole
- Ropinirole
- Selegiline
- Amantadine
- Anticholinergic agents.

These medications given in combination appear to have a much higher propensity to produce confusional psychosis.

Visual hallucinations are the most common clinical feature of drug-induced psychosis and are found in approximately 30% of treated patients. In most cases, hallucinations are nonthreatening and recurrent but can be threatening or frightening in approximately 28% of patients. Dysfunction of central serotonergic pathways has been suggested as a cause of drug-induced psychosis.

Management

Psychiatric symptoms in patients with PD and dementia are associated with behavioral, cognitive, and functional problems. Because hallucination is a significant risk factor for nursing home placement and subsequent mortality, effective management is of paramount importance.

Triggering events should be investigated in sudden-onset psychosis in a previously unaffected patient. Possible precipitating events include:

- Urinary and pulmonary infections
- Metabolic encephalopathy
- Cerebrovascular events
- Central nervous system space-occupying lesions.

The first step in management of drug-induced psychosis or hallucinations is to decrease or discontinue adjunctive therapy, including:

- Anticholinergics
- Amantadine
- Selegiline
- Dopamine agonists.

Decreasing the dose of levodopa should be attempted if psychosis continues. Unfortunately these measures can worsen parkinsonism.

If hallucinations and paranoia persist, the treating physician must consider a neuroleptic agent. Although all standard neuroleptics will worsen the motor manifestations of the disease, the atypical agent, clozapine (Clozaril), has been used successfully without aggravating the extrapyramidal state. In open studies, low dosages of one fourth tablet (6.25 mg), titrated to 25 mg to 100 mg/day (lower than those used to treat paranoid schizophrenia) have been shown to ameliorate psychoses in many patients.[16,17] The Parkinson Study Group is currently conducting a placebo-controlled trial of clozapine.

However, one such trial found that patients with marked dementia were less likely to respond to clozapine.[18] The difference was largely attributed to patients' inability to tolerate the clozapine's most common side effects, which are:

- Postural hypotension
- Sedation
- Delirium
- Sialorrhea.

Postural hypotension is discussed below. Patients ordinarily develop tolerance to clozapine's sedative effect; another stragety is to administer clozapine earlier in the evening. Sialorrhea can be controlled by suctioning.

Clozapine is also associated with some very serious adverse effects, with the most dangerous, fatal agranulocytosis, which necessitates weekly white blood cell monitoring of all patients taking it. In one published report of agranulocytosis in a PD patient, however, the process reversed and, therefore, was not fatal.[18]

Olanzapine (Zyprexa), a newly released atypical antipsychotic agent, is currently being evaluated in a multicenter, placebo-controlled trial involving patients with Parkinson's psychosis. No information is yet available on another newly released antipsychotic, quetiapine fumarate. Improvement of hallucinosis has also been reported with the serotonin-receptor antagonist, ondansetron, an antiemetic used in cancer patients.

■ **Sleep Disorders**

The earliest of the common sleep disturbances to be noted in PD patients is sleep fragmentation. Others include:[19]

- Vivid dreaming
- Nocturnal vocalization
- Excessive daytime sleepiness
- Altered sleep-awake cycles.

Compared with healthy, elderly subjects, parkinsonian patients have greater problems with sleep maintenance, although both have problems with sleep initiation. Daytime napping is more common in PD, as are problems with altered dreaming. A polysomnograph and video recording study of 12 Parkinson's patients with sleep disturbance showed CR carbidopa/levodopa to be more effective than the standard form in improving sleep efficiency, consolidation, and subjective evaluation. The improvement was not associated with improved motor function.

Although sleep disturbances appear to be related more to the underlying disease process than to antiparkinsonian medications, altered dreaming, nightmares, and vocalizations seem to be related to medications and generally precede hallucinations.

If patients become drowsy after each dose of medication, lowering the amount of the dose may be helpful. If the sleep-wake cycle is disturbed, a nighttime sedative at bedtime and a stimulant during the day may be necessary. The sedating antidepressants are also good soporifics, as are the benzodiazepines. For daytime stimulation, activity, caffeine, and, rarely, stimulants may be tried.

Orthostatic Hypotension

Many patients with PD suffer from orthostatic hypotension, caused either by the disease itself or by the medications used to treat it.[9] (When orthostatic hypotension is severe or is associated with other signs of autonomic dysfunction, such as disturbances of gastrointestinal motility and urinary bladder function, the possibility of multisystem atrophy or Shy-Drager syndrome should be considered.) Any of the antiparkinson medications can cause or exacerbate this symptom, although the direct dopaminergic agonists are the most likely.

Although orthostatic hypotension is characterized by a drop in blood pressure (BP), it is useful to consider it from the standpoint of its cause, decreased cerebral perfusion, since many patients with PD may have significant but asymptomatic drops in BP that do not warrant treatment. Moreover, not all patients with the symptom require treatment. If the light-headedness is minimal or brief, a few cautionary measures may suffice, including:

- Sit with the feet over the edge of the bed for a couple of minutes before getting up in the morning, then stand at the bedside for a while before walking away.
- Drink a large glass of water first thing in the morning.
- Do not limit fluid in the evening (even to avoid the late-night need to get up and urinate).
- Compression (at least 30 mm Hg to 40 mm Hg) of the lower extremities with special thigh-high stockings, although these may be too cumbersome for Parkinson's patients.

A number of pharmacologic agents are directed at increasing BP. They include the mineralocorticoids, which increase sodium reabsorption in the kidney. The resultant exchange with potassium introduces the risk of hypokalemia, however. Thus, prescribing or increasing a mineralocorticoid in patients with poor delivery of adequate sodium to the distal tubule is ineffective. In fact, a common mistake is the prescription of mineralocorticoids for patients on salt-restricted diets.

The mineralocorticoids are likely to take several weeks to become effective. A suggested dosing schedule of fludrocortisone (Florinef) is 0.2 mg/day, increased to 0.4 mg/day.

Ankle edema and weight gain are expected side effects of fludrocortisone. Patients should be watched for complications of the increased plasma volume, such as:

- Cardiac symptoms
- Symptoms of congestive heart failure
- Severe edema
- Supine hypertension.

Most patients do not need more powerful drugs. For those who do, however, a new α_1-adrenoreceptor agonist, midodrine (ProAmatine), is now available.[20] Midodrine is a prodrug, which, with its active metabolite desglymidodrine, produces increased vascular tone and an elevation in BP via activation of the α-adrenergic receptors of the arteriolar and venous vasculature. Desglymidodrine does not stimulate cardiac β-adrenergic receptors and diffuses poorly across the blood-brain barrier. Since midodrine is a prodrug, it is absorbed as a partially active compound, thus potentially reducing adverse gastrointestinal affects.

In a multicenter, randomized, placebo-controlled trial involving 162 patients with neurogenic orthostatic hypotension (19 with PD), 79 were treated with midodrine, 83 received placebo. Major end points were standing BP and symptoms of light-headedness, both of which were significantly improved.

The most noteworthy adverse events were:
- Piloerection (goosebumps, tingling, and itching, especially of the scalp) in 11 (13%) patients
- Urinary retention in five (6%) patients
- Supine hypertension, either *de novo* in three (4%) patients or increased in two (2%) patients.

Treatment of the supine hypertension includes elevation of the head of the bed and a flexible drug schedule. Given midodrine's duration of action of approximately 4 hours, patients may omit a dose if activities don't require standing for the next few hours, for example, and should not take it after 6 PM.

Dosage and administration of midodrine are:

- Starting dose: 2.5 mg at breakfast and lunch
- Increased by 2.5 mg increments daily with maximum 10 mg tid, q 4 hrs, on rising, mid-day and late afternoon
- Can be given at 3-hour intervals if needed but not more frequently.

Combined use of any of these antihypotensive drugs and antihypertensive agents is often ineffective, resulting in exacerbating both supine hypertension and orthostatic hypotension.[2]

Gastrointestinal Side Effects

Nausea is a recognized, relatively common side effect of all dopaminergic agents.[2] Taking carbidopa-levodopa with food is sometimes helpful. If this fails, addition of carbidopa in the form of a supplement (available from Dupont Pharma at no charge) is often effective in shunting levodopa into the brain. Should nausea remain a problem a peripheral dopamine blocking agent such as domperidone, which does not cross the blood-brain barrier, has been found to be extremely effective in reducing both nausea and postural hypotension. The drug is currently available only in Canada, Mexico, and Europe, however.

Autonomic dysfunction causing impaired gut motility is commonplace in PD. Constipation still remains one of the most frequent autonomic-related complaints throughout the disease process. The etiology is probably multifactorial, including:
- Lack of dietary fiber
- Inadequate fluid intake
- Diminished physical activity
- Aging
- Antiparkinson medications:
  - Levodopa
  - Dopamine agonists

- Anticholinergics
- Amantadine.

High-fiber diet, hydration, an exercise program, and regularly scheduled toileting are encouraged and must be tried initially. In addition:

- Anticholinergics and narcotic-containing compounds should be avoided.
- Bulk agents and laxatives can be prescribed. The stool softeners bran, psyllium, and docusates (up to 400 mg/day) are effective within 1 to 3 days; diphylmethane cathartics work within 6 to 8 hours; milk of magnesia is effective shortly after administration.
- Enemas may be effective in difficult cases.
- Prokinetic agents may be used to promote gastric emptying through enhancement of gut motility. Drugs that antagonize central dopamine receptors, such as metoclopramide (Reglan), should be avoided. Cisapride (Propulsid, 10 mg to 20 mg, tid, before meals), a relatively new parasympathomimetic agent, has been effective in gastroparesis and some types of constipation.

A recipe that has proved effective for many patients; mix 1 cup bran, 1 cup applesauce, 1 cup prune juice. Mixture can be refrigerated, but any unused portion should be discarded after 1 week. Take 2 Tbsp every morning, or mix 1 Tbsp of each ingredient every morning as needed.

1. Golbe LI, Sage JI. Medical treatment of Parkinson's disease. In: Kurlan R, ed. *Treatment of Movement Disorders.* Philadelphia, Pa: JB Lippincott Co; 1995:1-56.

2. Waters CH. Managing the late complications of Parkinson's disease. *Neurology.* 1997;49(1 suppl 1):S49-S57.

3. Fahn S. Parkinsonism. In: Rowland LP, ed. *Merritt's Textbook of Neurology.* 9th ed. Baltimore, Md: Williams & Wilkins; 1995:713-730.

4. Hurtig HI. Problems with current pharmacologic treatment of Parkinson's disease. *Exp Neurol.* 1997;144:10-16.

5. Nutt JG, Woodward WR, Hammerstad JP, Carter JH, Anderson JL. The "on-off" phenomenon in Parkinson's disease. Relation to levodopa absorption and transport. *N Engl J Med.* 1984;310:483-488.

6. Mouradian MM, Juncos JL, Fabbrini G, Schlegel J, Bartko JJ, Chase TN. Motor fluctuations in Parkinson's disease: central pathophysiological mechanisms, Part II. *Ann Neurol.* 1988;24:372-378.

7. Kurth MC. Using liquid levodopa in the treatment of Parkinson's disease. A practical guide. *Drugs Aging.* 1997; 10:332-340.

8. Luquin MR, Scipioni O, Vaamonde J, Gershanik O, Obeso JA. Levodopa-induced dyskinesias in Parkinson's disease: clinical and pharmacological classification. *Mov Disord.* 1992;7:117-124.

9. Waters CH. Management of patients with complicated Parkinson's disease. Syllabus, Course 127. American of Neurology Annual Meeting, Seattle, WA. 1995:33-42.

10. Riley DE, Lang AE. The spectrum of levodopa-related fluctuations in Parkinson's disease. *Neurology.* 1993;43:1459-1464.

11. Otani K, Mihara K, Okada M, Kaneko S, Fukushima Y. Crossover reaction between haloperidol and amoxapine for NMS. *Br J Psychiatry.* 1991;159:889. Letter.

9

12. Steur EN. Increase of Parkinson disability after fluoxetine medication. *Neurology.* 1993;43:211-213.

13. Montastruc JL, Fabre N, Blin O, Senard JM, Rascol O, Rascol A. Does fluoxetine aggravate Parkinson's disease? A pilot prospective study. *Mov Disord.* 1995;10:355-357. Letter.

14. Stern MB. Electroconvulsive therapy in untreated Parkinson's disease. *Mov Disord.* 1991;6:265. Letter.

15. Faber R, Trimble MR. Electroconvulsive therapy in Parkinson's disease and other movement disorders. *Mov Disord.* 1991;6:293-303.

16. Friedman JH, Lannon MC. Clozapine in the treatment of psychosis in Parkinson's disease. *Neurology.* 1989;39:1219-1221.

17. Lew MF, Waters CH. Clozapine treatment of parkinsonism with psychosis. *J Am Geriatr Soc.* 1993;41:669-671.

18. Greene P, Cote L, Fahn S. Treatment of drug-induced psychosis in Parkinson's disease with clozapine. *Adv Neurol.* 1993;60:703-706.

19. Nausieda PA, Leo GJ, Chesney D. Comparison of conventional and Sinemet CR on the sleep of parkinsonian patients. *Neurology.* 1994;44(suppl 2):A219. Abstract.

20. Low PA, Gilden JL, Freeman R, Sheng KN, McElligott MA. Efficacy of midodrine vs placebo in neurogenic orthostatic hypotension. A randomized, double-blind multicenter study. Midodrine Study Group. *JAMA.* 1997;277:1046-1051.

10 Nonpharmacologic Management of Parkinson's Disease

Nonpharmacologic therapy, essentially psychological support, is of incalculable value from diagnosis throughout the course of Parkinson's disease (PD).[1] Patients derive benefit from the knowledge that the disease is an area of active research and that increasingly effective medications and other interventions are on the horizon. Patients with careers and young families need realistic prognostic information, which often relieves excessive fears of early disability.

A suggested timetable for discussion of the disease and its implications for patients' future quality of life is seen in Table 10.1. Heritability is not discussed unless the patient has a positive family history since the hereditary pattern remains unclear and not amenable to genetic counseling.

Recommendation that patients join a support group is put off until initial stress of the diagnosis has passed and they are able to cope with seeing patients in more advanced stages of the disease. The timing of additional, more distressing topics, such as the probability of dementia, impotence, and incontinence is probably best left to the patient.

The comprehensive management of PD patients is a team effort involving a variety of therapeutic interventions and therapists, including the:[2]

- Primary physician
- Neurologist
- Family members
- Physical, occupational, speech therapists.

TABLE 10.1 — TOPICS FOR DISCUSSION EARLY IN COURSE OF PARKINSON'S DISEASE	
Approximate Timing	**Topics**
At diagnosis	• Outline general nature of PD and its treatability
After Diagnosis	
1-2 months	• Explain prognosis of typical case • Outline ongoing research related to prophylaxis and treatment • Recommend lay literature • Recommend joining national support societies • Follow-up re-reading, national support societies

8 months	• Educate regarding treatment complications to be aware of:
	  − Dose-related wearing-off
	  − Dyskinesia
	  − Mental difficulty

2 years	• Recommend joining local support group • Recommend regular exercise schedule, if patient is sedentary
Abbreviations: PD, Parkinson's disease.	
Adapted from: Golbe LI, Sage JI. In: Kurlan R, ed. *Treatment of Movement Disorders*. 1995.	

Although the diagnosis and management plan of PD and related movement disorders are largely handled by neurologists, family or primary physicians are frequently the first to be consulted by patients with early parkinsonian signs and symptoms. They are often the first to suspect the diagnosis and to refer patients to specialists and are likely to provide coordination of therapy thereafter.

Family members are regularly involved in care and as disability progresses, often become the primary caregivers, supported by home health-care nursing, physicians, and specialized therapists.

The primary physician, with the assistance of an occupational therapist, must assess limitations of the patient's daily activities as they occur. Activities to be evaluated regularly include:

- Grooming
- Dressing
- Walking
- Eating
- Washing dishes
- Playing cards
- Writing letters
- Reading the newspaper
- Housecleaning
- Making beds
- Cooking meals
- Gardening
- Driving.

Environmental Modifications

The first level of adaptation to PD centers around the patient's environment, which should be evaluated during a home visit by an occupational therapist. Patient and family should be questioned about:

- Door sills
- Scatter rugs
- Furniture in high traffic areas of the house
- Faucet and door handles that are difficult to use
- Other structural impediments to daily living.

Simple adaptations to these environmental barriers can be helpful in fostering an active existence.

Some specific modifications include:

- A bed low enough to allow the patient to rise easily
- A chair with arm rests and a firm seat to facilitate dressing
- A urinal or commode near the bed for night-time use
- If stiffness is a problem, a bed cradle made from a sturdy cardboard box will keep bed-clothes from entangling feet and lower legs when patient turns in bed
- A trapeze over head of the bed or a cord attached to the frame may help in changing positions or rising
- Button fasteners, zipper extensions, elastic shoe laces.

In the bathroom, the patient's life can be made simpler by:

- A raised toilet seat and a grab bar on the adjacent wall
- A toothpaste tube squeezer and a large-handled toothbrush
- An electric razor
- Tub and shower seats and grab bars
- Grooming aids in the shower, including a suction brush, soap on a rope, a sponge on a long handle.

In the kitchen, a number of adaptations can facilitate patients' daily lives, including:

- Utensils with large handles and knives that cut with rocking motion
- Combination utensils such as combined fork and spoon
- Easy-hold cups, flexible plastic straws, and nonskid plates

- Jar-lid openers
- Wooden reachers.

A few general, practical aids available from occupational therapists can also be recommended to help in the activities of daily living, including:
- A push-button telephone adapter with large keys to prevent misdialing
- Risers under the rear legs of straight-back chairs to help patient stand up (usually preferable to spring chairs or devices with wheels, which may be more dangerous than helpful)
- A book holder to help stabilize pages
- A special aid to stabilize a fingertip for typing or using the computer.

Driving

Driving may an integral part of the Parkinson patient's life and, therefore, may be a significant indication of his or her independence. Considerations in assessing driving ability should include:
- Judgment
- Mental status
- Reaction speed.

Side effects of medication must also be considered in this context. The tendency to freeze can be fatal. Since the decision regarding driving is always difficult, the most objective approach is to have the patient take an approved driver instruction course or retake the state driver's license test.

Patient Education

Many patient education resources are available from the various foundations and associations devoted to PD and from pharmaceutical companies (Table

10.2) Physicians recommending these materials should be familiar with their contents, however, since recommendation implies endorsement.

Physical Therapy

Walking 1 mile a day is often considered a reasonable goal, although many patients can walk much farther than that. Swimming is often recommended, especially for patients who swam earlier in life. It may also be useful for patients with asymmetrical disease, since it forces them to use the more affected side to swim in a straight line.

TABLE 10.2 — SELECTED PATIENT EDUCATION MATERIALS AND SOURCES

- **National Parkinson Foundation**
  - The Parkinson's Patient: What You and Your Family Should Know
  - Parkinsonian Handbook: Agenda for Parkinson Patients and Their Families
  - Nutritional Considerations of Parkinson's Disease

- **American Parkinson Disease Association**
  - Speech Problems and Swallowing Problems in Parkinson's Disease
  - Equipment and suggestions to help the patient with Parkinson's disease in the activities of daily living

- **Parkinson's Disease Foundation**
  - Exercise for the Parkinsonian Patient With Hints for Daily Living
  - Parkinson Patient at Home

- **United Parkinson Foundation**
  - Parkinson's Disease and the Young Patient
  - Parkinson's Disease: Glossary and Definitions

Reprinted with permission from: Goetz CG, et al. *Continuum.* 1995;1(4):115.

Patients who play golf, tennis, or racquetball or those who hike, bicycle, or jog should be encouraged to continue these activities on a regular basis. Others

---

FIGURE 10.1 — SELECTED EXERCISES WITH VERBAL CUES FOR THE PARKINSON'S DISEASE PATIENT

Back Thigh Stretches

This exercise is designed to reduce tightness and cramping in the back thigh muscles.

Position
Lie on your back with your knees bent. Arms are stretched above your head.

Action
- Raise your right knee.
- Stretch your heel toward the ceiling.
- Point your toes toward your nose.
- Bend your right knee and place it back at the start position.
- Repeat, raising the right knee.
- Stretch your heel toward the ceiling.
- Point your toes toward your nose.
- Do ten stretches, alternating legs.

Verbal Cues
"Try ten to really stretch your hamstring muscles."
"One... Right knee up, heel toward the ceiling, toes point to nose and down."
"Two... Left knee up, heel up, toes point to nose and down."
"Three... Right up, heel up, toes point, watch your leg, and down."
"Four... Left up, stretch your leg, point your toes, down."
"Five... Right, feel the stretch. Really stretch! Down."
"Six... Left, count along. You can do it! Good."
"Seven... Right knee up, heel up, toes point, and relax."
"Eight... Left, lift, now you have got it! Fine, lower."
"Nine... Right, raise that leg. Stretch the thigh and ankle, lower."
"Ten... Left, make this last one really count. Good! And, rest."

Continued

High-Step Marching

Marching while walking is designed to challenge you to lift your feet with every step and also loosens the hips.

Action

Bring your toes and knee up with every step you take. March as you walk.

Verbal Cues

"March with the music."
"March right, march left, and right, and left, lift toes, lift high. Good. Right, march left, march right, march left."
"Continue with the music and lift, and right, and left, right, left, right, left, right, left, return to your starting point and relax. Good."

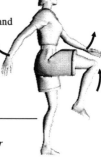

Arm X's and Y's

This exercise is helpful for your deep breathing and posture.

Position

Lie on your back. Your legs are straight, hands crossed and touching your upper thighs.

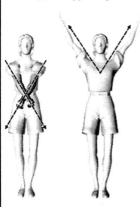

Action

- Spread your hands as you inhale and raise the arms over your head up and out to make a V.
- Make fists and exhale as you lower your arms across your hips making an X.
- Rest and repeat 10 times.
- At another time; sit in a straight chair with your wrists crossed on top of your knees.
- Perform this movement as above from the seated position.
- For more exertion, small hand weights may be used to increase your strength.

Verbal Cues

"Loosen your shoulders as well as improve your breathing. Count loudly for ten."

"One... Up, open your hands, inhale as you stretch up and out and make a V."

"Two... Down, exhale, closing your fists as you lower arms crossed to make an X."

"Three... Up, inhale, open hands, stretch up and out, over your head."

"Four... Down, exhale, make a fist, lower your arms down and across hips."

"Five... Way up now! Inhale deeply. Are you making a Y?"

"Six... Cross down, breathe all the way out, form an X."

"Seven... Up, make a V. Look at your hands as you stretch further. Good!"

"Eight... Down, cross the arms as you look down."

"Nine... Inhale and up. Look and count."

"Ten... Breathe out, and down. Fine and rest."

Shift, Lift and Step

*This exercise is helpful when you
need extra momentum to get unglued.*

Position

Stand straight with feet 6 inches apart. Hands open, arms at your sides. For extra safety stand in front of a chair.

Action

Shift your weight to your left leg as you lift your right toes and step forward on heel, then toes down.

Balance and step back.

Shift your right leg as you lift your left toes and step forward as before.

Balance and step back.

Do 10 times, alternating legs.

Verbal Cues

"Ready for ten."

"One... shift to left, right toes up and step forward... step back."

"Two... Shift to right, left toes up and step forward... then back."

"Three... Left, step, your arms relaxed... then back."

"Four... Right, step, feel your weight shift, good... then back."

"Five... Keep counting and shifting, toes up, step forward and rest."

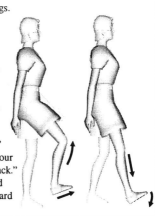

benefit from ballroom or square dancing. Some simple exercises that can be adapted for home use are illustrated in Figure 10.1.

As PD advances, most patients will benefit from formal physical therapy, which should be based on a needs assessment and specific goals. Prescribed exercises may improve the shuffling gait, stooped posture, and postural instability.

■ Tremor, Rigidity, Bradykinesia

Although these cardinal features of PD cannot be eliminated by nonpharmacologic approaches, their impact on patients' functional status can often be alleviated with physical and occupational therapy. In addition to the exercises described in Figure 10.1, a few additional simple ones may relieve functional disability due to rigidity and bradykinesia (Table 10.3).

Physical therapy may also help patients with rigidity and akinesia and disordered movement patterns. The approach involves practicing simple movements, such as touching typewriter keys before beginning more complex maneuvers. Patients may be taught to exaggerate movements by using a gross effort that extends too far and then, through practice, is refined into a smoother move. In this way, they can learn to handle faucets, doorknobs, and dressing and grooming activities. Lines painted on the floor can help patients step more regularly and may help to overcome freezing.

Symptoms of slowness and stiffness may be improved by repetitive movement exercises. First the involved joint is moved passively, later, actively with assistance, until eventually it can be controlled by the patient.

■ Gait Disturbance

This problem is related to primary motoric disturbances as well as impairment in the ability to perform asymmetrical muscle contraction of the trunk.

TABLE 10.3 — EXERCISES TO RELIEVE RIGIDITY AND BRADYKINESIA

- **Exercise to arise from chair**: Slide forward on the seat, leaning from the hips so that the body is at a 45° angle. Position one foot under the edge of the chair seat and the other foot one-half step forward. Next, position hands at the side of the seat near the front legs of the chair, and push with the arms while stepping forward, all in one continuous motion.

- **Exercise to sit down in a chair**: Reverse the process described for rising from the chair. Turn one's back to the chair, place one foot behind the other, bend the torso at a 45° angle, then sit slowly but smoothly while grasping the sides of the chair with the hands.

- **Exercise for stooped posture**: Stand with one's back to the wall, with the head, shoulders, buttocks, and heels all touching the wall. After holding the position for 30 seconds, walk away from the wall and then return, assuming the same position.

These exercises should be repeated 5 to 10 times every morning and evening to improve functional ability.

Reprinted with permission from: Goetz CG, et al. *Continuum.* 1995;1(4):121.

10

Patients have difficulty shifting weight from side to side. A focused approach to gait disorders involves particular attention to weight shifting, using exaggerated movements, to be practiced at home after initial instruction.

Hesitation when starting to walk (start hesitation) and the temporary inability to move (freezing) can sometimes be overcome by issuing verbal commands ("ready, set, go") to initiate movement and by learning to begin walking in a vigorous, sometimes marching fashion.

Patients with postural instability may begin walking with a few involuntary steps backward. Since these patients have a tendency to fall, their shoes should have leather, not rubber, soles and heel lifts to help tilt them forward.

Speech Therapy

A major source of disability in PD is disordered speech: hypophonia, dysarthria, and reduced variability in pitch and rhythm. Poor respiratory control also causes mumbled speech. Rigidity and bradykinesia involving the speech musculature aggravate all these problems.

Other dyskinesias that may impair communication include
- Tongue protrusion
- Lip smacking
- Grimacing
- Laryngeal stridor.

Although common late in the disease, speech and communications problems may appear early, particularly if the patient must speak at work. Thus, early speech therapy may be helpful.

Speech therapy emphasizes breathing control; patients practice augmentation of voice loudness and variation in pitch. Exercises are intended to increase the number of words spoken with each breath. Patients may also find that reading or singing aloud is a good practice exercise. Watching lip and tongue movements in mirror while speaking may help identify problems. A metronome may help patients to achieve measured speech.

Referral information regarding speech therapy for PD patients is available from the American Speech-Language-Hearing Association, 10801 Rockville Pike, Rockville, MD 20852. (301) 897-5700

Occupational Therapy

Occupational therapy may emphasize general activities of daily living or specific adaptations intended to keep the patient working. Employment may be the patient's usual premorbid occupation or a new type of work more appropriate for an individual with a movement disorder. Therapy usually includes exercises and other training to enhance fine motor coordination.

Many PD patients remain employed for a long time, often through making selective adaptations or job changes. A reading list of books by authors who have the disease is provided in Table 10.4 and may be useful to PD patients.

Psychotherapy

The psychological changes that affect PD patients can be more devastating than the motor impairment, particularly early in the disease. Moreover, emotional stress can increase motor symptoms. Physicians as well as family and friends should consider the context in which the disease usually occurs. At a time when most people are looking forward to retirement, financial independence, and increased enjoyment of life, the newly diagnosed Parkinson patient faces the prospect of progressive disability, physical dependence, and high medical costs.

Not surprisingly, the most common psychological problem faced by these patients is depression. Primary-care physicians caring for PD patients often find it helpful to all concerned to refer patients and their families to a psychological counselor experienced with the mental and emotional problems of the disease.

TABLE 10.4 — OCCUPATIONS AND AGE AT DIAGNOSIS OF AUTHORS WITH PARKINSON'S DISEASE

- **Carpenter, fireman, and poet**: Frank Ball. *These Parkinson Times*. Coventry, England: Aries Printers; 1989. Diagnosed at age 50.

- **Construction manager, photographer, journalist**: John R. Pierce. *Living With Parkinson's Disease*. Knoxville, Tenn: Spectrum Communications; 1989. Diagnosed in 1974 in his late 50s.

- **French professor**: Michael Monnot. *From Rage to Courage: The Road to Dignity Walk*. Northfield, Minn: St. Denis Press; 1988. Diagnosed in 1977 at age 38.

- **Home economics teacher**: Glenna W. Atwood. *Living Well With Parkinson's*. New York, NY: John Wiley; 1991. Diagnosed in 1981 at age 50.

- **Psychiatrist**: Cecil Todes. *Shadow Over My Brain*. Gloucestershire, England: The Windrush Press; 1990. Diagnosed in 1970 at age 39.

- **Sculptor**: Jan Peter Stern. *A Parkinson's Challenge: A Beginner's Guide to a Good Life in the Slow Lane*. 1987: 4th ed, 1991. Diagnosed in 1982 at age 55.

- **Teacher**: Eva B. Popper (wife of a Parkinson's disease patient). *My Love, My Care, My Spouse: A Chronicle of Parkinson's Disease*. Beltsville, Md: Parkinson Support Groups of America; 1988. Husband was diagnosed in 1973 at age 62.

Reprinted with permission from: Goetz CG, et al. *Continuum*. 1995;1(4):120.

Dental Care

Preventive measures are particularly important for patients diagnosed with PD because later diagnosis and treatment of dental disease becomes increasingly difficult.[3] A number of medications, including anticholinergics and antidepressants, commonly prescribed for Parkinson's patients cause xerostomia (dry mouth) by suppressing the production of saliva, thus reducing its antibacterial and cleansing actions, resulting in an increased risk for coronal and root surface caries, periodontal disease, and tongue erosion. Chemically induced xerostomia is sometimes employed to reduce drooling in patients with sialorrhea.

Saliva is also important because it dissolves food particles, thus allowing keener taste sensations, aiding digestion, and lubricating the food bolus for easier swallowing. It also lubricates oral tissues and facilitates clear speech.

The "on-off" phenomena, when associated with dyskinetic movements, twisting of trunk or limbs, and writhing of the tongue and lips, can pose problems for both patient and dentist. However, improved techniques and new restorative and prosthetic materials make it possible to perform procedures that were not feasible for these patients 2 decades ago.

Denture retention depends to a large extent on appropriate muscle function. Tremors or dyskinesias affecting the tongue may dislodge a mandibular denture and rigid and uncontrolled facial muscles may prevent the maxillary denture from maintaining a good retentive seal. Furthermore, elderly patients or those who have been edentulous for many years lack a bony ridge height for dentures to rest on, affecting the ability to keep them in place.

The use of local anesthesia is not contraindicated in patients with PD, although demerol probably should not be prescribed for patients taking selegiline since a rare interaction has been reported. Concomitant medical problems, such as heart disease and hypertension should be considered by dentists in planning treatment and anesthesia.

Levodopa was once thought to cause softening of tooth enamel and, in turn, an increased incidence

183

of caries. The increased tendency to tooth decay among Parkinson's patients is now thought to be the result of xerostomia and the decreased ability to perform regular oral hygiene.

New varieties of electric and sonic toothbrushes facilitate dental care for Parkinson patients. Flossing between teeth is made easier by floss holders. Optimum results require brushing the teeth with a fluoride and tartar-control dentifrice after meals and before retiring at night. Dilute fluoride rinses, such as neutral sodium fluoride solution or a stannous fluoride tablet dissolved in water, are sold without prescription and can be used daily as a one-minute rinse to protect the teeth. (The solution should not be swallowed.) In choosing a mouthwash, patients should avoid those that contain alcohol, which increases drying of the oral mucous membrane.

Family Counseling

Parkinson's disease has implications for virtually all facets of the family's life and future security.[2] Common family reactions include anger and concomitant guilt, depression, fatigue, and social isolation. Helping the family or caregivers to understand PD and what it must mean to the patient can be helpful. Some physicians keep a lending library of books on the disease for this purpose.

Family members or caregivers should be encouraged to accompany patients on physician visits. Support groups for patients and their families, which are widely available, provide patients with opportunities to share information about the disease and available services; about new books, therapies, and aids to daily living. Such groups also offer psychological support and sounding boards about the more troublesome aspects of the disease.

Physicians should help ensure that patients and their families are using all available community resources. Valuable sources of information include the leading national foundations devoted to PD, which provide newsletters, books, and general information regarding the disease (Table 10.5). Foundations can also guide patients and families to resources within their own communities.

Nonpharmacologic Approach to Associated Disorders

■ **Swallowing Problems and Sialorrhea**

These disorders may develop at any stage of PD and can be thoroughly evaluated by a speech therapist. Symptoms may include:

- Choking
- Coughing
- Drooling
- Holding food in the mouth.

Motor problems contributing to these difficulties include:

- Decreased tongue mobility
- Decreased elevation of the larynx
- Impaired swallowing reflex
- Diminished pharyngeal peristalsis.

Patients may fail to swallow saliva automatically, resulting in pooling in the mouth and throat. Saliva buildup may also contribute to muffled speech.

Careful attention to the process of swallowing may help improve sialorrhea and related problems. Patients should be advised to consciously swallow saliva frequently, with a studied movement of the saliva to the back of the throat before attempting to swallow. Holding the head upright helps to prevent

TABLE 10.5 — PARKINSON'S DISEASE FOUNDATIONS

- **National Parkinson Foundation, Inc.**
  1501 NW Ninth Avenue
  Bob Hope Road
  Miami, FL 33136-1494
  (800) 327-4545
  (800) 433-7022 in Florida
  (800) 522-8855 in California
  Website: www.parkinson.org

- **United Parkinson Foundation***
  833 W. Washington Boulevard
  Chicago, IL 60607
  (312) 733-1893

- **Parkinson's Disease Foundation***
  710 W. 168th Street
  New York, NY 10032-9982
  (212) 923-4700
  (800) 457-6676
  Website: www.parkinsons-foundation.org

- **American Parkinson's Disease Association, Inc.**
  1250 Hylan Boulevard, Suite 4B
  Staten Island, NY 10305
  (718) 981-8001
  (800) 223-2732
  Website: www.apdaparkinson.com

- **Parkinson Foundation of Canada**
  710-390 Bay Street
  Toronto, ON M5H 2Y2
  Canada
  (416) 366-0099
  (800) 565-3000 in Canada
  Fax: (416) 366-9190
  Website: www.parkinson.ca

* Merger negotiations in progress at press time.

pooling and enhances the swallowing mechanism. Finally, a conscious effort to swallow saliva must be made before speaking.

Patients should also think through each step of chewing and swallowing. They should eat slowly, taking only small amounts of food with each bite. Food should be chewed thoroughly and swallowed before the next bite is taken. Some patients may require video fluoroscopic evaluation of swallowing and, possibly, may need placement of a percutaneous esophagogastrostomy tube.

■ Nutritional Disturbances

Patients often have trouble preparing food, eating, or swallowing. In frustration, they may consume a very restricted diet, a problem enhanced by coexisting depression or dementia. Dietary consultation is often useful. However, certain general considerations can be emphasized by physicians, including:

- The diet should include all food groups
- Caloric intake should be sufficient to maintain body weight
- Include sufficient fiber and fluid to prevent constipation and enough calcium to avoid osteoporosis.

Specific dietary considerations for PD patients include:

- Because ingested protein may reduce the absorption of levodopa, meal planning and timing must be considered with the medication schedule in mind.
- Supplemental iron may also interfere with the action of carbidopa/levodopa; if it is necessary, timing of medications must be changed accordingly.
- Taking medications with meals may reduce drug absorption by simple bulk competition;

maximal absorption occurs when the stomach is empty.

■ Constipation

Both the inactivity inherent in PD and the drugs taken to control its manifestations can lead to constipation (see Chapter 9, *Complications of Parkinson's Disease and Its Therapy*). Gastrointestinal autonomic dysfunction may contribute as well. Management includes:

- Regular physical exercise
- Adequate intake of water and dietary fiber
- Use of stool softeners.

■ Seborrheic Dermatitis

Although the cause of seborrheic dermatitis and the reasons for its association with PD are unknown, effective therapies to provide symptomatic relief and control are available. Characterized by excessive sebum production by sebaceous glands and rapid skin cell turnover, seborrheic dermatitis leads to an inflammatory response that manifests as patchy or scaly, reddened, itchy skin. On the scalp, the condition may be simple dandruff or can involve the whole spectrum of signs and symptoms.

Although patients with PD tend to have long-term problems with seborrheic dermatitis, levodopa tends to resolve the condition or decrease its severity. The explanation seems to be that levodopa decreases sebaceous gland activity.

The condition can usually be treated with over-the-counter medications, including:

- Neutral or bland acne soap
- Ketoconazole shampoo
- Shampoos and lotions containing selenium (used as directed, 2 or 3 times a week, due to its ability to cause hair loss with excessive use)

- Shampoos, lotions, and creams containing pyrithione zinc.

Hydrocortisone and products with higher concentrations of selenium are available but require a physician's prescription. If the condition does not respond to nonprescription strategies, intermittent treatment with a prescribed product may be appropriate. Some dermatologists may prescribe antifungal agents.

■ Sexuality

Many otherwise normal individuals in their later decades have decreased sexual desire and function, as do many PD patients. Autonomic dysfunction with impotence, sleep disturbance, depression, and a general sense of fatigue in parkinsonism all take a toll on patients' sexuality. Exercise, adequate diet, and counseling to improve self-esteem can be helpful.

An honest and personal account of sex and PD, *In Sickness and in Health: Sex, Love and Chronic Illness* by Lucille Carlton, has been cited as filling a vast vacuum in the approach to the parkinsonian patient, specific advice on coping with disease, aging, and sexual diminishment.

Levodopa may induce feelings of well-being, and in some patients, results in a significant but generally short-lived increase in sexuality. Hypersexuality has also been described with dopamine agonist therapy. Such problems should be anticipated by both physician and family.

REFERENCES

1. Golbe LI, Sage JI. Medical treatment of Parkinson's disease. In: Kurlan R, ed. *Treatment of Movement Disorders.* Philadelphia, Pa: JB Lippincott Co; 1995:1-56.

2. Goetz CG, Jankovic J, Koller WC, Lieberman A, Taylor RB, Waters CH. Nonpharmacological approaches to the management of Parkinson's disease. *Continuum.* 1995;1(4):114-129.

3. Paulson RB, Paulson GW. Dental considerations for the Parkinson's patient. *Parkinson Report.* 1997;19:23-26.

11   Surgery

Surgical procedures for Parkinson's disease (PD) declined rapidly with the introduction of levodopa. Recently, however, interest in surgery has been rekindled as a result of problems with chronic levodopa treatment of this relentlessly progressive disease. Tremor is variably responsive to medication, many patients develop drug-associated motor fluctuations and dyskinesias, and symptoms that are not amenable to medication, such as postural instability and freezing, emerge over time.

In addition to and perhaps because of these shortcomings of medical intervention, there have been major advances in stereotactic surgery, including:

- Improved instrumentation with more precise target localization
- Computed tomography (CT)- and magnetic resonance imaging (MRI)-guided localization
- Intraoperative electrophysiologic monitoring and stimulation techniques that permit reversible disruption of neuronal function
- New awareness of functional anatomy resulting in identification of more rational targets
- Advances in transplant biology that suggest the possibility of implanting dopamine-producing cells.

A wide variety of neurosurgical operations have been proposed over the years for the treatment of PD, many of which are now obsolete. Currently the most popular techniques are:

- Thalamotomy
- Pallidotomy

- Chronic deep-brain stimulation (DBS) of the ventral intermediate (Vim) nucleus of the thalamus, subthalamic nucleus (STN), and globus pallidus internus (GPi), using an implantable pulse generator (IPG).

The basic technique of pallidal and thalamic surgery is similar.[1] Whether a lesion is to be made or DBS performed, the procedure is identical down to the point at which either a lesion is made or the stimulator implanted. The procedures are done using MRI guidance with the patient in the "off" state, under local anesthesia, and the Elekta Leksell G frame in place. The stereotactic three-dimensional coordinates of the anterior and posterior commissures are determined using the scanner's computer software. The desired target is chosen, its stereotactic coordinates read off, and the patient is taken to the operating room.

The bulk of the operating time is taken up in physiologic confirmation of the target site, using a microelectrode advanced to the selected target. Continuous recording or microstimulation every 1.0 mm is carried out along the trajectory, starting 10 mm to 15 mm above and extending a variable distance into or through the target[1] (Figure 11.1).[2] Up to 4 trajectories, 2 mm to 3 mm apart, and 6 trajectories, 2 mm apart, are usually sufficient in pallidal and thalamic exploration, respectively.

When a neuron is encountered, it is studied for any receptive field (RF) by applying tactile (hair-bending, light touch, deep pressure) or thermal stimuli, passive joint bending, muscle compression, auditory or visual stimuli, and by asking the patient to carry out voluntary movements on the contralateral side of the body. In the case of pallidal units, there may also be ipsilateral movement-related RFs. The locations of RFs are mapped out on body diagrams called figurine charts, visual responses on maps of the visual fields.

FIGURE 11.1 — PATTERNS OF NEURAL ACTIVITY WITHIN THE BASAL GANGLIA

A.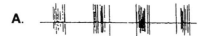

B.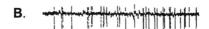

C.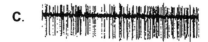

D.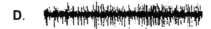

E.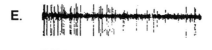

F.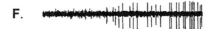

A. GPe intermittent high frequency first cell.
B. Typical irregular 30 to 60 Hertz firing of GPe cell.
C. Typical high frequency 150 to 500 Hertz discharge pattern of GPi.
D. Border cell.
E. Response of GPi cell to hip flexion (inhibition).
F. Response of GPi cell to hip flexion (excitation).

Abbreviations: GPe, globus pallidus externa; GPi, globus pallidus interna.

Photo courtesy of M. Dogali, MD.

Projected fields (PFs) are similarly mapped by determining the effects of threshold stimulation (up to 100 mA).

Pallidotomy done in this way requires 2 to 3 hours, thalamotomy 4 to 6 hours. One additional hour is necessary for insertion of a DBS electrode. The electrode's position may be confirmed with an image intensifier showing the tip at the location of the central beam in a sagittal view.

Deep-brain stimulation electrodes are attached to a temporary transcutaneous cable for short-term stimulation before internalization to insert a radio frequency-coupled, battery-powered, totally programmable IPG.

Pallidotomy

Modern pallidotomy is based on a prospective strategy aimed at restoring functional alterations in neuronal circuitry consequent to degeneration of dopamine neurons in the substantia nigra pars compacta (SNc) (Figure 11.2).[3]

In the 1950s, pallidotomy with a target site in the anterodorsal part of the pallidum became a popular procedure for PD. Thalamotomy soon replaced pallidotomy as procedure of choice, however, because it was believed to relieve tremor more consistently and to be associated with a lower rate of symptom recurrence. Tremor and rigidity were reported to recur in 25% of patients after pallidal surgery compared to only 11% after thalamotomy.

In 1992, posteroventral pallidotomy in 38 patients whose main complaint was hypokinesia was reported to produce long-lasting tremor relief, complete or almost complete relief of rigidity and hypokinesia and improvement in speech, gait, dystonia, and levodopa-induced dyskinesias.[4,5] But adverse effects included

FIGURE 11.2 — BASAL GANGLIA CIRCUITRY

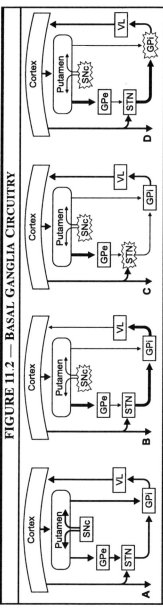

In normal basal ganglia circuitry, output from the gobus pallidus interna (GPi) exerts a chronic inhibitory effect on thalamocortical and brain stem neurons. Activation of the direct pathways inhibits firing of the GPi, whereas activation of the indirect pathway stimulates it. Dopamine from the substantia nigra pars compacta (SNc) stimulates the direct and inhibits the indirect pathway (a). In Parkinson's disease, loss of striatal dopamine secondary to degeneration of SNc neurons dimished inhibition of the GPi by the direct pathway and increases excitation of the GPi by the indirect connection. Increased GPi output results, in turn, in inhibition of thalamocortical and brain stem neurons (b). A lesion of the subthalamic nucleus (STN) diminishes the excessive excitatory stimulation of the GPi, consequently reducing the inhibitory outflow to brainstem and thalamocortical pathways (c). A lesion of the GPi directly diminishes its inhibitory output (d).

Adapted from: Hauser RA, et al. In: Kurlan R, ed. *Treatment of Movement Disorders*. 1995:57-93.

11

195

central homonymous visual field defects in 14% of patients and one instance of transitory facial weakness and dysphasia, reflections of damage to the optic tract and internal capsule, which lie in close proximity to the GPi.

Over the next few years, a number of new developments in stereotaxis, now routinely used, have resulted in reducing the originally 6- to 10-hour operation to 3 hours, and the early complications of visual impairment and hemiplegias have virtually been eliminated.[6] In 1995, 18 patients with medically intractable PD characterized by bradykinesia, rigidity, and marked "on-off" fluctuations underwent stereotactic ventral pallidotomy under local anesthesia. Targeting was aided by anatomic coordinates derived from the MRI, intraoperative cell recordings, and electrical stimulation before lesioning.

Assessment of motor function was made at baseline and at 3-month intervals for 1 year. Patients improved in bradykinesia, rigidity, resting tremor, and balance, with resolution of medication-induced contralateral dyskinesia. All quantifiable test scores after surgery improved significantly with patients off medications for 12 hours. Medication requirements were unchanged, but patients were able to tolerate larger doses because of reduced dyskinesia.

Finally, a recently published study of posterior GPi pallidotomy in 15 patients with medically intractable PD resulted in significant improvement of all cardinal parkinsonian motor signs as well as reduced drug-induced motor fluctuations and dyskinesias.[7] Improvement occurred predominantly contralateral to the lesion but was also present ipsilaterally. Mean total Unified Parkinson's Disease Rating Scale (UPDRS) and Schwab and England scores did not show a statistically significant decline over the 1-year postoperative period. Surgery resulted in little morbidity, including a lack of significant deficits on neuropsychological and psychiatric testing.

■ **Patient Selection**

Candidates for pallidotomy are patients with medically intractable PD as defined by significant motor morbidity not optimally managed by medication. Features responsive to pallidotomy are:

- Motor fluctuations
- "On-off" phenomenon
- Dystonia ("off" or "on")
- Drug-induced dyskinesia.

Additional criteria include:

- Demonstration of a clear and long-lasting benefit from antiparkinson medication, levodopa and dopamine agonists in particular
- Treatment of any existing depression
- Thorough assessment of patients' cognitive state. (Those with significant cognitive decline may be unable to cooperate with motor and visual field testing during the procedure and are less likely to have long-lasting improvement.)

Thalamotomy 11

Stereotactic thalamotomy was introduced in the 1950s, with lesions created with chemicals, heat, or freezing.[3] The procedure became a regular treatment for prominent unilateral tremor in PD. Follow-up studies were usually short-term and the majority were unblinded. However, in one blinded study, an evaluation of 17 patients in long-term follow-up (mean, 10.9 years after unilateral or subthalamotomy), investigators used videotapes and the UPDRS to compare tremor ipsilateral and contralateral to the side of surgery.[8] (A sign of long-term efficacy would be reversal of tremor side dominance.)

Tremor was found to be significantly less in the upper extremity contralateral to the operated side, indicating that stereotactic thalamotomy improved the absolute magnitude or ameliorated the rate of progression of tremor.

It seems clear that the procedure can improve contralateral tremor (45% to 92% of patients) and, to a lesser extent, rigidity (41% to 92%).[3] Bilateral thalamotomies are reported to improve tremor in 33% to 73% of patients and rigidity in 22% to 74%. Bradykinesia, postural instability, and ipsilateral tremor are not improved.

Complications of thalamotomy have included:

- Contralateral hemiparesis (0.5% to 26% of patients), can be minimized with modern stereotactic techniques and use of microelectrode recording
- Seizures (less than 1.3%)
- Paresthesias, usually of lips or fingers (1% to 3%)
- Uncommonly, ataxia, apraxia, hypotonia, abulia, gait disturbances
- Perioperative mortality (0.4% to 6%) usually due to hemorrhage at lesion site. Mortality in the modern era is expected to be less than 1%.

Bilateral thalamotomy is associated with a higher incidence of complications, including:

- Speech and swallowing problems, particularly in those with preoperative dysfunction
- Worsening of dysarthria in 29% of patients.

Modern stereotactic techniques and staged procedures have improved but not eliminated these complications.

■ Patient Selection

Thalamotomy, which has been found extremely effective in relieving parkinsonian tremor, rigidity, and drug-induced dyskinesia, has not generally been reported to be effective in alleviating akinesia and may even worsen gait or speech in some patients.[2]

However, in tremor-predominant patients, several points need to be considered:

- Thalamotomy is reportedly effective for tremor relief in 80% to 90% of patients compared to pallidotomy's more than 80%
- Thalamotomy patients have been studied in more detail and for longer periods
- Given the progressive nature of PD, patients' potential for developing other functionally disabling symptoms must be weighed against the likelihood and relative degree of improvement in tremor after thalamotomy versus pallidotomy.

Deep-Brain Stimulation

Chronic high-frequency thalamic stimulation has recently been described as an alternative to thalamotomy for the treatment of tremor in PD.[3] A stimulation frequency of 100 Hz to 250 Hz is generally employed, coupled with a pulse width of 60 to 210 microseconds. The current intensity or voltage necessary to alleviate tremor may increase progressively during the first months after surgery, presumably due to the development of fibrosis and increased resistance around the electrode tip, and must be adjusted accordingly. When stimulation is effective, tremor reduction occurs within 3 seconds, and the effect is lost within seconds of the stimulator being turned off. A rebound worsening lasting from a few minutes to several hours has been observed after discontinuation of chronic stimulation.

Previously used safely as a palliative for intractable pain related to somatosensory deafferentation and various movement disorders, chronic high-frequency thalamic stimulation was originally proposed as a less risky treatment than a second, contralateral procedure for patients with disabling tremor who had undergone a previous thalamotomy; if stimulation of the side opposite the original lesion caused complications, it could be turned off.

After the achievement of favorable results with combined thalamotomy and chronic thalamic stimulation for bilateral PD,[9] high-frequency thalamic stimulation was assessed as the initial surgical procedure in 26 patients.[10] Total suppression of contralateral tremor was observed in 68% of patients and major improvement in another 26%. A second study reported similar results, with total contralateral tremor suppression in 19 of 26 patients and improvement in the others.[11] Finally, a recently reported multicenter study of high-frequency, unilateral thalamic stimulation involved 29 patients with essential tremor and 24 with PD, 18 of whom had bilateral tremor.[12]

Stimulation was initiated 1 day postoperatively unless the patient exhibited a microthalamotomy effect (defined as tremor reduction with the IPG off, assumed to be due to the trauma of electrode placement). Patients were instructed on how to switch the device on and off with a hand-held magnet and to turn it off at night to preserve the battery and reduce the possibility of tolerance. Medication for PD (levodopa, 23 patients; dopamine agonists, 17; anticholinergics, 5) was held constant for at least 1 month before enrollment and during the first 3 months of the study.

Follow-up included a blinded evaluation 3 months after surgery with patients randomized to stimulation "on" or "off" and 6-, 9-, and 12-month open-label follow-up assessments. Evaluations consisted of:

- The UPDRS motor examination
- Global assessment of disability by both patient and examiner on a scale from 0 to 4
- Writing a sentence, drawing a spiral (see Chapter 4, *Etiology*), drawing a straight line between lines, pouring liquid
- Patients' subjective assessment of change from baseline to 3 months (marked, moderate, mild improvement, worsening, no change).

At the 3-month blinded evaluation and at 6-, 9-, and 12-month open label assessments results were:
- A significant decrease contralaterally in the clinical rating of tremor in stimulation "on" (Figure 11.3)
- Total resolution of their target tremors in 14 (58.3%) PD patients and 9 (31%) of those with essential tremor; one (4.2%) PD patient and one (3.4%) essential tremor patient had no change
- No effect observed in limb ipsilateral to the IPG
- Efficacy was not reduced at 1 year.

Complications related to surgery were few. Stimulation was associated with transient paresthesias lasting several seconds, which occurred in most patients at 3 months (Table 11.1). Complications related to the device that occurred during the first year were:
- Incisional skin infection, two patients, successfully treated with antibiotics
- IPG malfunction necessitating replacement, one patient
- Extension wire erosion necessitating replacement, one patient.

Beneficial effects have been noted through 5-year follow-ups of the early trials.[3] Although not studied in a systematic way, chronic stimulation may also im-

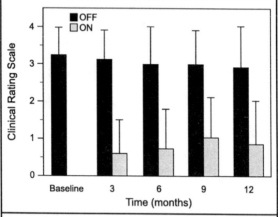

FIGURE 11.3 — CHANGE IN PARKINSONIAN TREMOR WITH CHRONIC THALAMIC STIMULATION

Shown here are blinded, clinical ratings of tremor at 3 months and open-label evaluations at 6, 9, and 12 months in Parkinson's disease patients with implantable pulse generators (IPGs) switched to "on."

From: Koller W, et al. *Ann Neurol*. 1997;42:292-299.

prove rigidity, unilateral pain, and dyskinesia. Akinesia appears to be unchanged. Adverse effects (paresthesias, dystonia, gait disorders, dysarthria) have been mild and generally resolve when stimulation is discontinued.

The principle advantage of thalamic stimulation is its potential to provide functional benefit without the creation of an irreversible lesion, particularly important in patients who are:

- Older
- With bilateral tremor
- Who have undergone an earlier contralateral thalamotomy
- With a pre-existing speech disorder.

TABLE 11.1 — COMPLICATIONS RELATED TO CHRONIC THALAMIC STIMULATION

Adverse Event	Months		
	3	6	12
Paresthesia	42 (79.2%)	19 (35.8%)	11 (20.8%)
Headache	6 (11.3%)	1 (1.9%)	2 (3.8%)
Disequilibrium	5 (9.4%)	3 (5.7%)	2 (3.8%)
Paresis (contralateral limb)	4 (7.6%)	2 (3.8%)	2 (3.8%)
Gait disorder	3 (5.7%)	1 (1.9%)	0 (0.0%)
Dystonia	3 (5.7%)	1 (1.9%)	2 (3.8%)
Dysarthria	2 (3.8%)	1 (1.9%)	2 (3.8%)
Localized pain	1 (1.9%)	0 (0.0%)	1 (1.9%)

Adapted from: Koller W, et al. *Ann Neurol.* 1997;42:292-299.

The procedure's principle disadvantages include:
- Possibility system will need replacement because of fracture or infection
- Battery requires replacement after several years. (May be obviated by development of externally rechargeable stimulators).

Although the mechanism of action of electrical stimulation of the Vim is not known, it may:
- Create functional ablation of a "firing center" or
- Serve to desynchronize abnormal depolarizations that have become overactive and autonomous.

Deep-brain stimulators have more recently been implanted in the GPi and STN to treat other motor signs of PD.[2] Both have been reported to improve all of the cardinal motor symptoms, including tremor.

However, stimulation in the STN has also been reported to induce dyskinesias at higher current intensities. Larger patient populations in well-controlled studies will be required to assess the benefits and improve the understanding of chronic DBS.

The effects of GPi stimulation on parkinsonian motor signs may be mediated by mechanisms similar to those proposed for thalamic stimulation. Assuming the improvement is a result of decreased GPi output, it can be the result either through inhibition or blocking of neuronal activity:

- Directly via depolarization block or
- Indirectly via antidromic activation of globus pallidus externa (GPe).

Similarly, STN stimulation has a host of possible mechanisms that underlie its beneficial effects on parkinsonian motor signs, including:

- Direct inactivation
- Indirect inactivation by alteration of GPi neuronal activity (decreasing it, blocking its transmission, or normalizing its pattern)
- Antidromic activation of GPe leading to inhibition of STN, GPi, and/or reticularis neurons in thalamus, leading, in turn, to normalization of thalamic neuronal activity.

Thus, the mechanism(s) underlying the effect of electrical stimulation in these subcortical structures are probably multifactorial, dependent on stimulation parameters and location of the stimulating electrode. Other sites where electrical stimulation may prove equally or more effective have yet to be explored. Acute stimulation within the GPe of patients undergoing pallidotomy reportedly improves bradykinesia. Given the many projections of the GPe to thalamus, GPi, and STN, which project in turn throughout the basal ganglia and beyond, normalization of activity within it would theoretically have a greater effect on amelioration of motor signs than stimulation of less far-ranging output areas.

Transplantation of Dopamine-Producing Cells

Because the principal pathological changes of PD are relatively isolated and involve specific degeneration of the dopaminergic nigrostriatal neurons, investigators have used several strategies to pursue the feasibility of replacing dying cells with an alternative vital population. For the past 15 years, clinical trials to evaluate the efficacy of intrastriatal dopamine transplants have been conducted.[13] Two donor tissues have been used:

- Chromaffin cells of the adrenal medulla
- Fetal nigral neurons of the ventral mesencephalon.

■ Adrenal Medulla Grafts

Adrenal chromaffin cell transplants, even with cografts of sural nerve, (a cellular source of trophic factors, including nerve growth factor), have proved disappointing, given the modest clinical benefits achieved and the significant morbidity associated with adrenal removal in fragile PD patients.

■ Fetal Nigral Transplantation

From a scientific perspective, fetal nigral grafts have been the most consistent and best donor cell for transplantation. Their use clinically was delayed, for the most part, by social and ethical concerns. And trials were hindered in the United States by a Presidential ban on National Institutes of Health (NIH) funding. Recently, however, clinical trials have been initiated.

Transplant Material

Fetal mesencephalic cells can be transplanted as either a cell suspension, used in most studied to date, or solid grafts.[14] Cell suspension grafts provide more homogeneous tissue distribution but necessitate pooling of tissue, and infection or rejection in any one donor could adversely affect all graft deposits. Solid grafts, on the other hand have an extended donor window, are easier to prepare, and preserve cytoarchitectural relationships. The preparations have shown comparable survival.

Implantation Site

Grafts may be implanted into the putamen, caudate, or both.[14] The postcommissural putamen is considered a good primary site for several reasons, including:

- Both autopsy and positron emission tomography (PET) scan studies demonstrate greater dopamine depletion within the posterior putamen than in the anterior putamen-caudate nucleus complex in Parkinson's patients
- Degeneration of the SNc in PD preferentially occurs in regions that project to the posterior putamen
- Experiments in methylphenyltetrahydropyridine (MPTP)-lesioned primates demonstrate that dopamine grafts placed exclusively into the putamen induce significant improvement of motor function.

The anterior putamen-caudate nucleus may also be an important target, however, because:

- Hemiparkinsonism can be induced by MPTP injection into the caudate nucleus
- Fetal nigral grafts placed into the caudate nucleus of MPTP-treated monkeys can induce significant functional recovery, with benefits

different from those associated with grafting into the posterior putamen.

The best clinical results may ultimately be associated with grafting into both caudate and putamen or into other potential target areas, such as the SNc and the nucleus accumbens.

Immunosuppression

Although immunosuppression is not essential in the immunologically privileged central nervous system, surgical trauma or the graft itself could disrupt the blood-brain barrier and permit the immune system access to graft antigens.[14] Thus, most transplant groups treat study patients with cyclosporin A (CsA) for varying periods before and after the procedure. The absence of evidence of immune rejection 1 year after discontinuation of CsA has suggested that prolonged immunosuppression may not be necessary. In any case, the need for immunosuppression after fetal transplantation remains controversial.

Patient Selection

Identification of the best candidates for a neural transplantation procedure is not yet established.[13] Currently, the only justifiable criterion is the presence of advanced PD that cannot be satisfactorily controlled with available medical therapy. However, these patients have greater perioperative risk, as well as signs and symptoms that do not respond to levodopa, thus they may not be capable of responding to grafted dopaminergic neurons. Such problems may be less significant in patients with early disease, who also may not require drug therapy, thereby avoiding issues relating to the potential toxic effects of levodopa metabolites on graft viability.

Clinical Findings

Worldwide, an estimated 200 patients with PD have received implants of embryonic mesencephalic tissue into the striatum.[15] In 13 patients (two with MPTP-induced parkinsonism), PET documented increased fluorodopa uptake in the grafted striatum compared to preoperative levels. This finding indicates that grafted dopamine neurons can survive and grow in the human parkinsonian brain. Moreover, autopsy findings in two patients who died from unrelated events 18 and 19 months, respectively, after transplantation strengthened this hypothesis by revealing robust survival of transplanted neurons, with reinnervation of the postcommissural putamen.[13]

Results have been inconsistent and difficult to compare, however, because of:

- Variations in patient selection
- Transplant variables
- Rating systems
- Level of scrutiny
- Clinical expertise.

Selected examples are summarized in Table 11.2.[14-21]

The most recently reported trial involved six patients followed for 10 to 72 months after mesencephalic tissue from four to seven aborted human embryos (aged 6 to 8 weeks postconception) was grafted unilaterally into the putamen (four patients) or putamen and caudate (two).[15] According to the results of this study:

- Transplantation of embryonic mesencephalic tissue leads to survival of dopaminergic neurons with high reproducibility.
- Unilateral intrastriatal grafts can induce therapeutically valuable improvement in a majority of graft recipients.

				Donor				Benefit				% ↓	F-D
Reference	No. of Patients	CsA	Type of Transplant	Age (PC, weeks)	No. of Donors	Bilateral Grafts	Site	N	ML	MD	MK	L-dopa	PET
Lindvall et al[16]	2	Yes	Suspension	7-9	4	No	Anterior P+C	0	2	0	0	0	
Lindvall et al[17]	2	Yes	Suspension	6-7	4	No	P	0	0	2	0	0	+
Freed et al[18]	2	4 of 7	Solid	5-6	1	No	C+P	1	0	1	0	39	
	5		Solid	5-6	1	Yes	P	0	2	3	0		
Spencer et al[19]	4	Yes	Solid	5-9	1	No	C	1	3	0	0	24	−
Widner et al[20]	2	Yes	Suspension	6-8	6-8	Yes	C+P	0	0	0	2		+
Freeman et al[21]	4	Yes	Solid	6.5-9	6-8	Yes	Posterior P	0	0	2	2	0	++
Wenning et al[15]	4	Yes	Solid	6-8	4-5	No	P	0	1	3	0	10-20	++
	2	Yes	Solid		5-7	No	C+P	0	1	1	0		++

TABLE 11.2 — PUBLISHED OUTCOMES OF FETAL TRANSPLANTATION

Abbreviations: CsA, cyclosporin A; C, caudate; N, none; ML, mild; MD, moderate; MK, marked; F-D PET, fluorodopa uptake on positron emission tomography; −, no benefit; +, increased uptake; ++, markedly increased uptake.

Adapted from: Olanow CW, et al. In : Watts RL, Koller WC, eds. *Movement Disorders: Neurologic Principles and Practice.* 1997.

11

- Grafts can restore putaminal fluorodopa uptake to a normal level.
- Functional recovery is incomplete and variable, possibly related to variable survival and reinnervation by graft, differences between patients in dopaminergic denervation pattern, and other brain pathology.
- Despite evidence of long-term graft survival (up to 6 years) continuing degeneration of patients' own dopamine systems could still limit the graft-derived improvement.
- Complete bilateral grafting is necessary for optimal long-term functional recovery.

Despite these positive findings, many investigators have found a subnormal pattern of innervation, and surviving dopaminergic neurons still represented a small fraction (5% to 10%) of the original population of grafted cells.[14] Clearly, all transplantation trials for PD remain experimental.[15] Thus, all such procedures should be performed only by groups with laboratory transplant experience and expertise in tissue dissection, stereotactic surgery, PD, and clinical trials.

Improvement of neurite outgrowth from grafted dopamine neurons might be achieved by the exposure of grafts, either *in vitro* or *in vivo*, to trophic factors, such as:

- Brain-derived neurotrophic factor (BDNF)
- Basic-fibroblast growth factor (BFGF)
- Glial-derived neurotrophic factor (GDNF).

Both BDNF and GDNF have been shown to enhance neurite outgrowth from fetal nigral neurons and GDNF promotes graft survival in rodent models of PD.

Future Directions

The entrance of molecular biology into the field of neural transplantation has led to exciting advances, which greatly extend the ability to manipulate and generate cell lines that may be candidates for transplantation in PD and may ultimately supplant fetal grafting.[13,14] Among the major new approaches to direct delivery of therapeutic agents into the central nervous system are:

- Polymer encapsulated cells
- *Ex vivo* and *in vivo* gene therapy
- Implantation of immortalized cells engineered to produce a specific protein.

■ Polymer Encapsulated Secreting Cells

The encapsulation process uses either polyelectrolyte-based microcapsules or thermoplastic-based macrocapsules, which can contain:

- Adrenal chromaffin tissue
- Dopamine-producing tumor lines
- Cells genetically engineered to release GDNF.[22]

Surgical implantation of dopamine-producing tumor cells (PC12) has been associated with behavioral improvement in motor function in parkinsonian animals.

The capsules are designed to selectively allow the diffusion of smaller neuroactive molecules, such as dopamine, and restrict the entrance of large antibody molecules, thus theoretically preventing immunologic reactions even if the transplanted tissue is of foreign origin. However, encapsulated cells cannot reinnervate the host brain and are limited to providing diffusible substances to the immediately surrounding brain parenchyma.

■ *Ex Vivo* Gene Therapy Using Autologous Cells

In this hypothetical scenario, a PD patient's own cells (generally fibroblasts) are genetically modified to express tyrosine hydroxylase (TH), then are grafted into appropriate sites in the striatum to provide a local supply of levodopa at sites in the brain normally innervated by dopaminergic neurons.[23] The levodopa secreted by these cells may then be taken up by remaining neuronal and nonneuronal cells, converted to dopamine, and released in either a normally regulated or unregulated fashion. Grafted into MPTP-treated monkeys, autologous fibroblasts were found to express TH for up to 4 months.

■ *In Vivo* Gene Transfer

Several vehicles have been used for *in vivo* transfer of cDNA sequences, including:[23]
- Herpes simplex viral vectors
- Adenoviral vectors
- Direct plasmid DNA transfer
- Lentivirus vectors.

A relatively new system uses adeno-associated virus (AAV), a human parvovirus, which, in addition to having no known pathology in man, is incapable of replication without helper function provided by adenovirus. Gene delivery vectors derived from AAV do not harbor any viral genes, thus lack the chromosome targeting of the wild-type virus. However, in recent studies, it has become apparent that AAV vectors can transduce a variety of tissue targets *in vivo* and gene expression can persist for periods of at least 18 months. Introduction of AAV vectors expressing β-galactosidase or TH into monkey brains resulted in detection of gene expression, restricted to the striatum, at 21 days and 3 months.

Further technological advances are required to optimize gene delivery, regulation of gene expression, and testing in appropriate functional models before gene therapy can be considered for treating human disease.

■ Implantation of Immortalized Cells

In this procedure, ventral mesencephalons are dissected from embryonic day 13 rats and dopaminergic cells are infected with the simian virus (SV 40) large T antigen, which renders them immortal at 33° C but permanently amitotic at 38° to 39° C.[14] Once the cells are transfected, clonal lines of dopamine-producing cells can be established, resulting in a limitless supply of neuronal-like progenitors, all of which express TH and synthesize dopamine.

Although results of early studies indicate that grafting of genetically modified neurons is encouraging, a number of fundamental issues still need to be resolved before this approach can be considered for clinical use.

REFERENCES

1. Tasker RR, Lang AE, Lozano AM. Pallidal and thalamic surgery for Parkinson's disease. *Exp Neurol.* 1997;144:35-40.

2. Vitek JL. Stereotaxic surgery and deep brain stimulation for Parkinson's disease and movement disorders. In: Watts RL, Koller WC, eds. *Movement Disorders: Neurologic Principles and Practice.* New York, NY: McGraw-Hill; 1997:238-255.

3. Hauser RA, Freeman TB, Olanow CW. Surgical therapies for Parkinson's disease. In: Kurlan R, ed. *Treatment of Movement Disorders.* Philadelphia, Pa: JB Lippincott Co; 1995:57-93.

4. Laitinen LV, Bergenheim AT, Hariz MI. Leksell's posteroventral pallidotomy in the treatment of Parkinson's disease. *J Neurosurg.* 1992;76:53-61.

5. Laitinen LV, Bergenheim AT, Hariz MI. Ventroposterolateral pallidotomy can abolish all parkinsonian symptoms. *Stereotact Funct Neurosurg.* 1992;58:14-21.

6. Dogali M, Fazzini E, Kolodny E, et al. Stereotactic ventral pallidotomy for Parkinson's disease. *Neurology.* 1995;45:753-761.

7. Baron MS, Vitek JL, Bakay RA, et al. Treatment of advanced Parkinson's disease by posterior GPi pallidotomy: 1-year results of a pilot study. *Ann Neurol.* 1996;40:355-366.

8. Diederich N, Goetz CG, Stebbins GT, et al. Blinded evaluation confirms long-term asymmetric effect of unilateral thalamotomy or subthalamotomy on tremor in Parkinson's disease. *Neurology.* 1992;42:1311-1314.

9. Benabid AL, Pollak P, Louveau A, Henry S, de Rougemont J. Combined (thalamotomy and stimulation) stereotactic surgery of the VIM thalamic nucleus for bilateral Parkinson disease. *Appl Neurophysiol.* 1987;50:344-346.

10. Benabid AL, Pollak P, Gervason C, et al. Long-term suppression of tremor by chronic stimulation of the ventral intermediate thalamic nucleus. *Lancet.* 1991;337:403-406.

11. Blond S, Caparros-Lefebvre D, Parker F, et al. Control of tremor and involuntary movement disorders by chronic stereotactic stimulation of the ventral intermediate thalamic nucleus. *J Neurosurg.* 1992;77:62-68.

12. Koller W, Pahwa R, Busenbark K, et al. High-frequency unilateral thalamic stimulation in the treatment of essential and Parkinsonian tremor. *Ann Neurol.* 1997;42:292-299.

13. Kordower JH, Goetz CG, Freeman TB, Olanow CW. Dopaminergic transplants in patients with Parkinson's disease: neuroanatomical correlates of clinical recovery. *Exp Neurol.* 1997;144:41-46.

14. Olanow CW, Freeman TB, Kordower JH. Transplantation strategies for Parkinson's disease. In: Watts RL, Koller WC, eds. *Movement Disorders: Neurologic Principles and Practice.* New York, NY: McGraw-Hill; 1997:221-236.

15. Wenning GK, Odin P, Morrish P, et al. Short- and long-term survival and function of unilateral intrastriatal dopaminergic grafts in Parkinson's disease. *Ann Neurol.* 1997;42:95-107.

16. Lindvall O, Rehncrona S, Brundin P, et al. Human fetal dopamine neurons grafted into the striatum in two patients with severe Parkinson's disease. A detailed account of methodology and 6 month follow-up. *Arch Neurol.* 1989;46:615-631.

17. Lindvall O, Brundin P, Widner H, et al. Grafts of fetal dopamine neurons survive and improve motor function in Parkinson's disease. *Science.* 1990;247:574-577.

18. Freed CR, Breeze RE, Rosenberg NL, et al. Survival of implanted fetal dopamine cells and neurologic improvement 12 to 46 months after transplantation for Parkinson's disease. *N Engl J Med.* 1992;327:1549-1555.

19. Spencer DD, Robbins RJ, Naftolin F, et al. Unilateral transplantation of human fetal mesencephalic tissue into the caudate nucleus of patients with Parkinson's disease. *N Engl J Med.* 1992;327:1541-1548.

20. Widner H, Tetrud J, Rehncrona S, et al. Bilateral fetal mesencephalic grafting in two patients with parkinsonism induced by 1-methyl-4-phenyl-1,2,3,6-tetrahydropyridine (MPTP). *N Engl J Med.* 1992;327:1556-1563.

21. Freeman TB, Olanow CW, Hauser RA, et al. Bilateral fetal nigral transplantation into the postcommissural putamen in Parkinson's disease. *Ann Neurol.* 1995;38:379-388.

22. Tresco PA, Winn SR, Aebischer P. Polymer encapsulated neurotransmitter secreting cells. Potential treatment for Parkinson's disease. *ASAIO J.* 1992;38:17-23.

23. Bankiewicz KS, Leff SE, Nagy D, et al. Practical aspects of the development of *ex vivo* and *in vivo* gene therapy for Parkinson's disease. *Exp Neurol.* 1997;144:147-156.

Note: Page numbers in *italics* indicate figures;
page numbers followed by t indicate tables.

Acquired immune deficiency syndrome (AIDS), 12t
Activities of daily living, rating of, 75t-76t, 83t
Adenoviral vector, 212
Adrenal medulla cells, transplantation of, 205
Adriamycin (doxorubicin), 68t
Age/aging
  anticholinergics and, 94
  dopamine agonist therapy and, 102
  genetic factors and, 24-25
  incidence and, 17
  motor fluctuations and, 21
  occupations and, at disease onset, 182t
  pharmacotherapy and, 88, *89*, 90
  posture and, 21
  preventive vitamin E and, 99-100
  selegiline monotherapy and, 98
  striatonigral neuron loss and, 23-24, *25-26*
  tremors and, 21
    essential, 60, 61t
Akinesia. See also *Bradykinesia.*
  freezing as, 153
Alcohol intake, 61t
Alien hand, 15
Alzheimer's disease, 13t, 15
  dementia in, 43, 66
    vs Parkinson's dementia, 156
  iron uptake and storage in, 50
  α-synuclein and, 25
Amantadine (Symmetrel)
  action mechanism of, 94-95
  dosage of, 93t, 95
  effectiveness of, 95
  indications for, *89*
  side effects of, 95, 155t, 159-160
Amino acids, excitatory, 52-53, 135
α-Amino-3-hydroxy-5-methyl-4-isoxasolpropionate (AMPA)
    receptor, 52-53
Amiodarone, 66, 68t
Amoxapine (Asendin), 158
AMPA receptor. See α-*Amino-3-hydroxy-5-methyl-4-*
    isoxasolpropionate receptor.
Amphotericin B, 68t
β-Amyloid, 49

Amyotrophic lateral sclerosis, 13t, 15
    causative toxin in, 27-28
Anergic (hypokinetic) depression, 58, 64
Anesthesia, local, 183
Anorexia, rating scale of, 81t
Anticholinergics. See also specific drug.
    contraindications to, 157
    dental care and, 183
    dosage of, 91t
    in elderly patients, 94
    indications for, *89*, 90, 94
    response to, 69t
    side effects of, 94, 155t, 159-160, 166
    trazadone similarity to, 157
Antidepressants. See also *Monoamine oxidase (MAO) inhibitors*.
    dental care and, 183
    indications for, 155t, 157-158
    side effects of, 157
Antiemetics, 14
Antioxidants, 98. See also *Oxidative stress*; *Oxygen free radicals*.
Antipsychotic drugs, 14
Anxiety attack, 154
Apomorphine, 159
Apoptosis
    bel-2 blockade of, 46
    in neurodegeneration, 48-49
Aricept (donepezil), 157
Arm swing, 58
Artane (trihexyphenidyl), 91t, 94
Ascorbate, 46
Asendin (amoxapine), 158
Aspiration pneumonia, 21
Atrophy, in multiple systems. See *Multiple system atrophy*.
Autonomic dysfunction, 58, 59t
    causes of, 165-166
    in multiple system atrophy, 64
    in parkinsonism-plus syndromes vs Parkinson's disease, 65t
    sexuality and, 189
Axial dystonia, 64
    in parkinsonism-plus syndromes vs Parkinson's disease, 65t

Babinski sign, 58
Basal ganglia
    anatomy of, 31, *32-33*, 33
    automatic reflexes and, 38
    calcification of, 15
    circuitry of, *195*
    degeneration of, 13t, 15

12

Basal ganglia (*continued*)
  iron content in, 71
  neural activity patterns in, *193*
  neurotransmitter balance in, 36-38, *37*
  in parkinsonism pathogenesis, 31, *32-34*, 33, 35-38, *37*
  pathways to and within, 33, *34*, 35-36
Bed, turning in and adjusting sheets in, 76t
Behavioral disorders, 154-162, 155t
bel-2 gene, 46
Benzamide, 67t
Benzisoxazole, 67t
Benzodiazepine, 155t
Benztropine (Cogentin), 91t, 94
Bethanechol, 68t
Binswanger's disease, 12t
  differential diagnosis of, 58, 62
Blepharospasm, 59t
L-BMAA (β-N-methylamino-L-alanine)
  action mechanism of, 50-51
  toxicity of, 27-28
Boxer, punch drunk, 14-15
Bradykinesia
  in drug-induced parkinsonism, 66
  in essential tremor, 61t
  in parkinsonism-plus syndromes, 65t
  in Parkinson's disease, 11, 57, 61t, 65t
  physical therapy for, 178-180, 179t
  rating of, 79t
  striatonigral degeneration and, 63
Brain
  oxidative stress vulnerability of, 46
  stimulation of. See *Deep-brain stimulation.*
Brain-derived neurotrophic factor, 210
Bromocriptine (Parlodel)
  dosage of, 91t, 102-103
  indications for, 102
  pramipexole effectiveness vs, 109
  ropinirole effectiveness vs, 111, *113*
  side effects of, 103, 115, 159
Bulbar palsy, spastic (Binswanger's disease), 12t
  differential diagnosis of, 58, 62
Butyrophenones, 67t

Calcium channel blockers, 68t
Carbidopa/levodopa (Sinemet). See also *Levodopa.*
  action mechanism of, 88
  clinical studies of, 131-134
  controlled-release, 131, 149, 155t
  dosage of, 92t, 130, 132

Carbidopa/levodopa (Sinemet). (*continued*)
  reason for combination of, 127
  remacemide and, 134
  selegiline as adjunct to, 96, 99, *100*
  side effects of, 130-131, 165
Carbon disulfide intoxication, 12t, 27
Carbon monoxide intoxication, 12t, 27
Catechol-O-methyltransferase (COMT) inhibitors. See also
    Entacapone (Comtan); *Tolcapone (Tasmar)*.
  action mechanism of, 88, 116
  dopamine and, 38
  dosage of, 93t
  indications for, *89*, 149
  for wearing-off phenomenon, 149
Caudate nucleus, 31, *32*
Cephaloridine, 68t
Cerebellar dysfunction, 65t
Ceroid-lipofuscinosis, 13t
Cheese effect, 98
Child, parkinsonism in, 17. See also *Age/aging*.
Chlorpromazine (thorazine), 67t
Chlorprothixene (Taractan), 67t
Cinnarizine, 12t, 68t
Cisapride, 152
Cisapride (Propulsid), 166
Classification
  of parkinsonism, 11, 12t-13t
  of Parkinson's disease, 20-21
Clinical Global Impression Scale, 111-112, *114*
Clozapine (Clozaril), 67t
  for psychosis, 155t, 160
  side effects of, 160-161
Cogentin (benztropine), 91t, 94
Cogwheel rigidity, 11, 68
Cogwheel rigity. See also *Rigidity*.
Compazine (prochlorperazine), 67t
Complications of Parkinson's disease and treatment
  behavioral/psychiatric disorders as, 154-162, 155t
  drug failure as, 152
  dyskinesias as, 150-152
  gastrointestinal, 165-166, 188
  immobility-related, 21
  internal tremor as, 141
  levodopa-related, 141-154. See also *Levodopa, side effects of*.
  nutritional disturbances as, 187-188
  on-off fluctuations as, *148*, 149-150
  orthostatic hypertension as, 162-165
  rating scales of, 80t-81t
  restlessness as, 141

12

Complications of Parkinson's disease and treatment (*continued*)
  seborrheic dermatitis as, 188-189
  sleep disorders as. See *Sleep disorders.*
  swallowing dysfunction as, 59t, 75t, 185, 187
Computed tomography (CT), surgery guided by, 191
Computed tomotraphy (CT). See also *Single photon emission
    computed tomography (SPECT).*
COMT inhibitors. See *Catechol-O-methyltransferase (COMT)
    inhibitors.*
Comtan. See *Entacapone (Comtan).*
Confusion, levodopa-related, 154
Constipation, 165-166, 188
Copper metabolism, 15
Cortical diffuse Lewy body disease, 13t
Cortical ganglionic degeneration, 13t, 15
Counseling, for family, 184-185
Coxsackie virus, 14
Cranial structures, changes in, 59t
Creutzfeldt-Jakob disease, 12t
Cyanide, 12t, 27
Cycad flour toxicity, 27-28

Daytime sleepiness, 155t, 161-162
Death from Parkinson's disease
  causes of, 21
  before levodopa, 19, 128
  with levodopa alone vs levodopa and selegiline, *100*
Deep-brain stimulation
  action mechanisms in, 204-205
  complications of, 201-202, 203t
  disadvantages of, 203
  effectiveness of, 200-201, *202*, 203-204
  patient selection for, 202
  techniques in, 199
Dementia, 13t, 15
  causes of, reversible, 156
  cortical, 156
  diffuse Lewy body disease and, 43
  in disease classification, 21
  early, 58, 155
  incidence of, 155
  medications in, 156-157
  neuroimaging in, 156
  in parkinsonism-plus syndromes vs Parkinson's disease, 65t
  Parkinson's vs Alzheimer's, 156
  progressive, 15
  rating scale of, 74t
  subcortical, 156
  thalamic, 13t

Demerol, selegiline interaction with, 183
Dental care, 182-184
Deprenyl and Tocopherol Antioxidative Therapy of Parkinsonism
    (DATATOP)
  clinical study from, on selegiline as neuroprotectant, 96, 98
  rating scale from, 19
Depression
  anergic (hypokinetic), 58, 64
  disease duration and, 157
  incidence of, 157
  pathophysiology of, 157
  rating scale of, 74t
  treatment of. See *Antidepressants*; *Monoamine oxidase (MAO)*
      inhibitors.
    electroconvulsive, 158
    psychotherapy in, 181
Dermatitis, seborrheic, 188-189
Desglymidodrine, 164
Diabetes mellitus, 28
Diagnosis of Parkinson's disease, 11, 13
  anergic depression vs, 58, 64
  Binswanger's disease vs, 58, 62
  characteristic tetrad (TRAP) in, 11, 13
  clinically possible, probable, or definite in, 57-58
  differential, 58-69
  drug-induced parkinsonism vs, 66, 67t-69t, 68-69
  essential tremor vs, 58, 60, *60*, 61t
  initial presentation in, 57
  laboratory findings in, 68, 70
  motor symptoms of, 59t
  multiple system atrophy vs, 58, 63-64
  neuroimaging in, 70-72
  nonmotor symptoms of, 59t
  normal-pressure hydrocephalus vs, 58, 62
  parkinsonism-plus diseases vs, 65t
  in prediagnostic period, 57
  striatonigral degeneration vs, 58, 63
Diazepam, 68t
Dibenzodiazepine, 67t
Dibenzoxazepine, 67t
Digital impedance, 58
Dihydroindolone, 67t
L-3,4-Dihydroxyphenylalanine. See *Levodopa.*
Diltiazem, 12t
Disulfiram, 12t
DLBD (diffuse Lewy body disease). See *Lewy body disease,*
    diffuse (DLBL).
DNA laddering, 48
DNA transfer, 212

12

Domperidone, 115-116, 165
  for drug failure response to levodopa, 152
Donepezil (Aricept), 157
Dopamine. See also *Levodopa.*
  activation of, 37
  depletion of, 12t, 14
  homovanillic acid from, 38
  inactivation of
    free radical formation and, 46
    by MAO inhibitor, 38, 46
  iron level and, 50
  neurotransmitter balance and, 36, *37*, 38
  nigrostriatal pathway of, 36, *37*
    destruction of, 14, *26*
  pars compacta and, 33
  storage of, 143
  synthesis of, 38
    compensatory, 54
  turnover of, 54
Dopamine agonists, 9, 101-116. See also specific drug, eg,
    Bromocriptine (Parlodel).
  action mechanism of, 88, 101
  age and, 102
  alone or with levodopa, 102
  dosage of, 91t-92t
  dyskinesia and, 101-102, 151-152
  indications for, *89*
  for on-off fluctuations, 150
  pharmacokinetics of, 101-102
  sexuality and, 189
  side effects of, 160
Dopamine receptors
  blockers of, 12t, 14
    brain compensating mechanisms and, *20*
  mRNA of, as marker of Parkinson's disease, 70
  pharmacologic profile and distribution of, 40
Dopamine-producing cell transplantation
  donor tissues for, 205-206
  effectiveness of, 208, 209t, 210
  immunosuppression in, 207
  implantation site for, 206-207
  patient selection for, 207
  from tumor, 211
  using immortalized cells, 213
Dopaminergic cells, loss of, 54
Dopaminergic neuron, 38, *39*
Down-gaze palsy
  in multiple system atrophy, 64
  in progressive supranuclear palsy, 62

Doxorubicin (Adriamycin), 68t
Dreaming, 154, 155t, 161-162
Dressing ability, 75t
Driving of vehicle, 173
Droperidol (Fentanyl), 67t
Drug therapy for Parkinson's disease, 61t, 65t. See also specific drug.
  age and, 88, *89*, 90
  amantadine in, *89*, 93t, 94-95
  anticholinergics in, *89*, 90, 91t, 94
  COMT inhibitors in. See *Catechol-O-methyltransferase (COMT) inhibitors.*
  dopamine agonists in. See *Dopamine agonists.*
  gastrointestinal disorders from, 165-166
  history of, 87-88
  levodopa in. See *Levodopa.*
  selegiline in, 93t
  timing of, 90
  vitamin E in, 99-100
Drug-induced parkinsonism, 12t, 14, 26-28
  agents causing, 66, 67t-68t
  differential diagnosis of, 66, 68, 69t
Dysautonomia, 15
Dyskinesia. See also *Wearing-off phenomenon.*
  causes of, 150
  diphasic, 151-152
  dopamine agonists and, 101-102
  levodopa-induced, 128, 150-152, 152t
  pathophysiology of, 101-102
  rating scales of, 80t
  symptoms of, 151, 152t
  threshold of, 143
  treatment of, *89*, 151-152
Dysphagia (swallowing dysfunction), 59t, 75t
  treatment of, 185, 187
Dystonia, 59t, 80t

Education of patient, 173-174, 174t
Effexor (venlafaxine), 157
Eldepryl (selegiline). See *Selegiline (Eldepryl).*
Elderly patients. See also *Age/aging.*
  anticholinergics for, 94
Electroconvulsive therapy, 158
Embolism, pulmonary, 21
Encephalitis lethargica, 13-14
Encephalitis/encephalopathy, parkinsonism after, 12t, 13-15, 62
Entacapone (Comtan). See also *Catechol-O-methyltransferase (COMT) inhibitors.*
  action mechanism of, 120, 122
  dosage of, 93t, 126t

12

Entacapone (Comtan). (*continued*)
  as levodopa adjunct, 122-125, *123-124*
  pharmacokinetics of, 126t
  side effects of, 126, 126t
  wearing-off phenomenon and, 125
Environment and etiology
  of parkinsonism, 11, 12t
  of Parkinson's disease, 26-28
Environmental modification, in home, 171-173
Epidemiology of Parkinson's disease, 9, 17
Essential tremor. See *Tremor, essential.*
Etiology
  of parkinsonism, 11, 12t
    drugs in, 12t, 14
    encephalopathy in, 12t, 13-14
    environment in, 11, 12t
    genetics in, 15
    idiopathic, 12t
    trauma in, 12t, 14
  of Parkinson's disease
    aging in, 23-24, *25-26*
    environment in, 26-28
    genetics in, 24-26
Etrafon (perphenazine and amitriptyline), 67t
Excitatory amino acids, 52-53, 135
Exercises, *175-177*
Experimental parkinsonism, 27
Extrapyramidal system, 31, *32*
Eye blinking, 58, 59t

Facial expression, 59t, 77t
Falling
  levodopa-related, 153
  unrelated to freezing, 76t
Familial disease. See also *Heredofamilial disease.*
  olivopontocerebellar atrophy as, 13t, 15
Family of patient, 171
  counseling for, 184-185
Febrile illness, 13
Fentanyl (droperidol), 67t
Ferritin, iron binding by, 46, 49
Fetal nigral transplantation, 205-206, 210
Fibroblast growth factor, basic, 210
Filipino X-linked dystonia-parkinson, 13t
Fingertip dexterity, 78t
Fludrocortisone (Florinef), 163-164
Flunarizine, 12t, 68t
5-Fluorouracil, 68t
Fluoxetine (Prozac), 68t, 157-158

Fluphenazine (Prolixin), 67t
Food cutting and utensil handling, scale of, 75t
Foot, dystonia of, 59t
Free radicals. See *Oxygen free radicals.*
Freezing, 153
  driving ability and, 173
Fungal infection, 12t

Gait
  axial structures and, 59t
  changes in, 20
    age and, 21
  freezing in, 153
  physical therapy for, 178-180
  rating scale of, 76t, 79t
Ganglionic degeneration, cortical, 13t, 15
Gastric emptying, 142
Gastrointestinal side effects
  pathophysiology of, 165-166
  treatment of, 166
Gaze palsy, 15, 65t
Gender, Parkinson's disease and, 17
Gene therapy, 9
  autologous, 212
Gene transfer, *in vivo*, 212-213
Genetics in disease pathophysiology. See *Heredofamilial disease.*
Gerstmann-Strausler-Scheinker disease, 13t
Glial-derived neurotrophic factor, 210
Globus pallidus
  anatomy of, 32
  environmental toxins and, 27
Glutamate transmission, 36, *37*, 135
Glutathione
  mitochondrial injury and, 51-52
  oxidative stress and, 45-48
Grasp reflex, 58
Guamanian Parkinson's disease-dementia-amyotrophic lateral
sclerosis, 13t, 15
  causative toxin in, 27-28

Hallervorden-Spatz disease, 13t, 15
Hallucinations
  levodopa-related, 159
  predisposing characteristics for, 158
  treatment of, 155t
  visual, 87, 154, 159
Haloperidol (Haldol), 67t
Hands
  dexterity of, 78t
  tremor of, 77t

12

Handwriting, scale of, *60*, 75t
Hemiatrophy-hemiparkinsonism, 12t
Hepatocerebral degeneration, chronic, 12t
Heredofamilial disease
  discussion topics in, timing of, 169
  essential tremor as, 60, 61t
  parkinsonism as, 13t, 15, 17
  Parkinson's disease as, 24-26
Herpes simplex viral vector, in gene transfer, 212
History of parkinsonism, 11, 13, 19
Hoehn and Yahr staging, 81t, 107
Home of patient, modifications in, 171-173
Huntington's disease, 13t, 15, 17
  differential diagnosis of, 63
  glutathione level in, 47
  iron uptake and storage in, 50
Hyaline inclusion disease, intracytoplasmic, 12t
Hydrocephalus, 12t
  normal-pressure, 58, 62
Hygiene scale, 76t
Hypersomnolence. See *Sleep disorders*.
Hypertension, supine, 164
Hypocalcemic parkinsonism, 12t
Hypokinetic (anergic) depression, 58, 64
Hypotension, orthostatic
  causes of, 162
  drugs for, 163-165
  prevention of, 163
Hypoxia, 12t

Immobility, complications from, 21
Immortalized cells, implantation of, 213
Immunosuppression, 207
Incidence of Parkinson's disease, 9, 17
Infarction, parkinsonism after, 12t
Infectious parkinsonism, 12t
Inherited degenerative disorders. See *Heredodegenerative disease*.
Insomnia. See *Sleep disorders*.
Intellectual impairment, 74t
Iron
  in Alzheimer's disease, 50
  in basal ganglia tissue, 71
  dopamine level and, 50
  peripheral metabolism of, 50
  protein binding of, 46
  striatonigral degeneration and, 49-50
Ischemia, apoptosis and, 49

Japanese B virus, 14
  parkinsonism after, 62
Juvenile parkinsonism, 17

Kainate receptor, 52-53
Kemadrin (procyclidine), 91t, 94

Laryngeal stridor, 15
Latency, of parkinsonism, 14
Laxatives, 166
L-BMAA (β-N-methylamino-L-alanine)
  action mechanism of, 50-51
  toxicity of, 27-28
Legs. See also *Lower extremities*.
  agility of, 78t
  restlessness in, 153-154
Lentivirus vectors, in gene transfer, 212
Lesions
  corticospinal, 58
  in Parkinson's disease, 41-43, *42-43*
Levodopa, 61t, 65t. See also *Carbidopa/levodopa*; *Dopamine*.
  beginning-of-dose deterioration and, 152
  controlled-release, 149
  delaying therapy with, 127
  dosage of, 92t
    motor fluctuations related to, 141-154
  drug failure response to, 152
  duration of therapy with, 128
  effectiveness of, 87
    long-term, 143, *144*
  entacapone with, 122-125, *123-124*
  for essential tremor, 61t
  ethyl ester of, 134
    remacemide with, 135
  future of, 9
  glutathione changes and, 47-48
  history of, 87
  indications for, *89*, 90
  in liquid form, 150, 152
  MPTP-induced parkinsonism and, 128
  for multiple system atrophy, 64
  oxidative stress and, 127
  for parkinsonism-plus syndromes, 65t
  Parkinson's disease mortality and, 19
  pharmacokinetics of, 87, 127, 141-144, 142t
  pramipexole with, 106, *108*
  prognosis and, 128
  ropinirole alone vs, 111, *112*
  ropinirole with, 112-115, *114*

12

Levodopa (*continued*)
  selegiline with, 96, 99, *100*
  sexuality and, 189
  side effects of
    age and, 90
    anxiety attacks as, 154
    beginning-of-dose deterioration as, 152-153
    burning pain as, 153
    drug duration and timing and, 127
    drug failure as, 152
    dyskinesias as, 87, 150-152, 152t
    falling as, 153
    freezing as, 153
    gait difficulties as, 154
    memory loss and confusion as, 154
    motor fluctuations as, 153-154
    on-off shifts as, 87, 149-150, 154
    pharmacokinetics and, 141-144, 142t
    restless legs as, 153-154
    timetable for, *145*
    treatment of, 146t, 148, 155t
    urinary, 154
    visual hallucinations as, 87, 154
    vocalizations as, 154, 155t
    wearing-off phenomenon as, 146t, 146-149, *147*
  for striatonigral degeneration, 63
Levodopa (*continued*)
  tolcapone with, 116-119, *118*
  toxicity of, 128-130
Levoprome (methotrimeprazine), 67t
Lewy bodies
  age and, 23
  in experimental parkinsonism, 27
  levodopa toxicity and, 129
  in striatonigral degeneration, 63
  structure of, 42-43, *43*
Lewy body disease, diffuse (DLBD), 42-43, *43*
  classification of, 43
  cortical, 13t, 15
  differential diagnosis of, 66, 156
Lithium, 12t, 68t
Lower extremities
  agility of, rating scales of, 78t
  changes in, 59t
  dystonia of, 151
  in Parkinson's disease vs essential tremor, 61t
  restlessness in, levodopa-related, 153-154
Loxapine (Loxitane), 67t
Lubag disease (Filipino X-linked dystonia-parkinson), 13t

Lytico-Bodig (Guamanian Parkinson's disease-dementia-
    amyotrophic lateral sclerosis), 13t, 15
  causative toxin in, 27-28

Machado-Joseph disease, 13t
Magnetic resonance imaging (MRI)
  in diagnosis of Parkinson's disease, 70-71
  surgery guided by, 191
Manganese intoxication, 12t, 27
MAO inhibitors. See *Monoamine oxidase (MAO) inhibitors.*
Markers of Parkinson's disease, 70
Melanin, neuronal vulnerability and, 54
Mellaril (thioridazine), 67t
Meperidine, 68t
Mesoridazine (Serentil), 67t
Methotrimeprazine (Levoprome), 67t
β-N-Methylamino-L-alanine (L-BMAA)
  action mechanism of, 50-51
  toxicity of, 27-28
N-Methyl-D-aspartate (NMDA) receptor
  neurotoxicity initiated by, 52-53
  remacemide and, 134-135
α-Methyldopa, 68t
Methylphenylpyridinium ion (MPP+)
  action mechanism of, 52
  mitochondrial injury and, 50
  neuronal toxicity of, 27
1-Methyl-4-phenyl-1,2,3,6-tetrahydropyridine (MPTP)
  action mechanism of, 50
  intoxication from, 12t, 14
    levodopa and, 128
    MAO inhibitors and, 27, 96
  remacemide and, 134
Metoclopromide (Reglan)
  contraindications to, 166
  indications for, 66
  parkinsonism from, 67t
Meyerson sign, 58
Micrographia, 59t
Midodrine (ProAmatine), 164-165
Mineralocoids, 163-164
Mirapex. See *Pramipexole (Mirapex).*
Mitochondrial cystopathy, 13t
Molindone (Moban), 67t
Monoamine oxidase (MAO) inhibitors. See also *Antidepressants*;
    Selegiline (Eldepryl).
  action mechanism of, 88
  dopamine inactivation by, 38, 46
  MPTP intoxication and, 27, 96

12

Motivation/initiative, rating scale of, 74t
Motor fluctuations, levodopa-related. See Levodopa, *side effects of.*
Motor neuron disease, 13t
MPP⁺. See *Methylphenylpyridinium ion (MPP⁺).*
MPTP. See *1-Methyl-4-phenyl-1,2,3,6-tetrahydropyridine (MPTP).*
Multiple system atrophy
  clinical features of, 63-64
  differential diagnosis of, 64, 65t
  glutathione level in, 47
  iron uptake and storage in, 50
  progression of, 64
  syndromes involving, 13t

Nausea/vomiting, 81t
Navane (thiothixene), 67t
Necrosis, apoptosis vs, 48-49
Nefazodone (Serzone), 158
Neuroacanthocytosis, 13t
Neurodegenerative disease
  apoptosis in, 48-49
  iron uptake and storage in, 49-50
  melanin and, 54
  nitrosoureas in, 28
Neuroimaging
  in diagnosis of Parkinson's disease, 70-72
  in Parkinson's vs Alzheimer's dementia, 156
Neuroleptics, 12t
  indications for, 66, 160-161
  parkinsonism from, 66, 67t
Neuromelanin, 33
  as free iron buffer, 49-50
Neuromelanin-containing neurons, degeneration of, 41, *42*
Neuronal plasticity, 25
Neuroprotection, 9, 87
  by remacemide, 135
  by selegiline, 96-98
Neurotoxicity, receptors triggering, 52-53
Neurotransmitters
  balance of, in normal and dopamine-depleted brain, 36, *37*, 38
  manipulation of, 9
Neurotrophic factors, 210
Nigral transplantation, from fetus, 205-206, 210
Nigrostrial degeneration. See *Striatonigral degeneration.*
Nitrosoureas, in diabetes mellitus and neurodegenerative
    diseases, 28
NMDA receptor. See *N-Methyl-D-aspartate (NMDA) receptor.*
β-N-Methylamino-L-alanine (L-BMAA)
  action mechanism of, 50-51
  toxicity of, 27-28

N-Methyl-D-aspartate (NMDA) receptor
  neurotoxicity initiated by, 52-53
  remacemide and, 134-135
Norepinephrine, freezing and, 153
Norzine (thiethylperazine), 67t
Nuchal dystonia, in parkinsonism-plus syndromes vs Parkinson's
  disease, 65t
Nutritional disturbances, 187-188

Occupational therapy, 171-173, 181, 182t
Olanzapine (Zyprexa), 67t, 155t, 161
Olivopontocerebellar atrophy
  differential diagnosis of, 65t
  familial, 13t, 15
  sporadic, 13t
  in striatonigral degeneration, 63-64
Oncovin (vincristine), 68t
On-off fluctuations
  causes of, 149
  dental care and, 183
  treatment of, 150, 154
Orthostasis, 81t
Orthostatic hypotension
  causes of, 162
  drugs for, 163-165
  prevention of, 163
Oxidative stress
  excitatory amino acids and, 52-53
  levodopa and, 127
  mechanics of, 45-48
  in parkinsonism, evidence against, 53-54
  selegiline monotherapy and, 98
Oxygen free radicals
  defense mechanisms against, 46
  levodopa and, 127
  as marker of Parkinson's disease, 70
  neurodegenerative disorders and, 46

p53 gene, 48
Pain, levodopa-related, 153
Pallidal atrophy, 13t
Pallidotomy
  advances in, 196
  basal ganglia circuitry and, *195*
  effectiveness of, 194, 196-197
  patient selection for, 197
  techniques in, 192, 194
Panencephalitis, subacute sclerosing, 12t
Paralysis agitans, 11

12

Parkinsonism
classification of, 11, 12t-13t
drug-induced, 12t, 14, 26-28
agents causing, 66, 67t-68t, 68
differential diagnosis of, 66, 68, 69t
experimental, 27
heredodegenerative, 13t, 15, 17
latency of, 14
parkinsonism-plus syndromes and, 13t, 15
pathophysiology of, 11
postencephalic, 12t, 13-14
incidence of, 62
pugilistic encephalopathy and, 14-15
secondary, 12t, 13-15
vs Parkinson's disease, 11, 12t
Parkinsonism-plus syndromes, 13t, 15. See also specific
syndrome, eg, *Supranuclear palsy, progressive.*
differential diagnosis of, 65t, 72
levodopa for, 65t
multiple system atrophy as, 63-64
progressive supranuclear palsy as, 62-63
single photon emission computed tomography of, 72
striatonigral degeneration as, 63
Parkinson's disease, natural history of. See *Progression of
Parkinson's disease.*
Parkinson's Disease foundations, 186t
Parkinson's disease-dementia-amyotrophic lateral sclerosis
(PD-D-ALS), 13t, 15
Parlodel. See *Bromocriptine (Parlodel).*
Paroxetine (Paxil), 157
Pars compacta, *32*, 33
Pars reticulata, 31, *32*
Parvovirus, in gene transfer, 212
Pathophysiology of Parkinson's disease, 11
apoptosis in, 48-49
basal ganglia in, 31, *32-34*, 33, 35-38, *37*
dopamine in, 38, *39*, 40-41
excitatory amino acids and, 52-53, 135
glutathione depletion in, 45-48
iron uptake and storage in, 49-50
Lewy bodies in, 42-43, *43*
mitochondrial injury in, 50-52
oxidative stress in, 45-48
evidence against, 53-54
respiratory chain activity in, 51
subthalamic nucleus in, 134
Patient education, 173-174, 174t
Paxil (paroxetine), 157
PD-D-ALS (Parkinson's disease-dementia-amyotrophic lateral
sclerosis), 13t, 15

Pergolide (Permax)
  dosage of, 92t, 104
  effectiveness of, 103-104
  indications for, 103
  pharmacokinetics of, 104
  side effects of, 104-105, 159
Permax. See *Pergodine (Permax)*.
Perphenazine (Trilafon), 67t
Perphenazine and amitriptyline (Etrafon, Triavil), 67t
Phenelzine, 68t
Phenergan (promethazine), 67t
Phenothiazines, 67t
Physical therapy, 174-175
  exercises in, *175-177*
  for gait disturbance, 178-180
  for tremor, rigidity, and bradykinesia, 178, 179t
Pick's disease, 13t
Pill-rolling tremor, 68
Platelets
  abnormalities in, as marker of Parkinson's disease, 70
  mitochondrial function in, 51
Pneumonia, aspiration, 21
Polymer-encapsulated dopamine-secreting cells, 211
Positron emission tomography (PET)
  in diagnosis of Parkinson's disease, 71-72
  in Parkinson's vs Alzheimer's dementia, 156
  in transplantation of dopamine-producing cells, 206
Postencephalic parkinsonism, 12t, 13-15
  incidence of, 62
Postural hypotension, 161
Posture, 11, 20, 57
  age and, 21
  in essential tremor, 61t
  instability of, levodopa-related, 153
  in parkinsonism-plus syndromes vs Parkinson's disease, 65t
  rating of, 79t
Pramipexole (Mirapex)
  adjunctive, 106, *108*, 109
  clinical trials using, 105-107, 109
  dosage of, 92t, 104, 106, 109, 110t
  indications for, 105, 109 110
  as monotherapy, 105-106
  side effects of, 106, 110, 159
  wearing-off phenomenon with, 106-107
Primary physician
  activity evaluations by, 170-171
  referrals to psychotherapist by, 181
Primidone
  for essential tremor, 61t
  for Parkinson's disease, 61t

12

ProAmatine (midodrine), 164-165
Procaine, 68t
Prochlorperazine (Compazine), 67t
Procyclidine (Kemadrin), 91t, 94
Progression of Parkinson's disease, 19-21, *20*
    vs drug-induced parkinsonism, 69t
    vs essential tremor, 61t
Progressive supranuclear palsy. See *Supranuclear palsy, progressive.*
    glutathione level in, 47
Prolixin (fluphenazine), 67t
Promazine (Sparine), 67t
Promethazine (Phenergan), 67t
Propranolol
    for essential tremor, 61t
    for Parkinson's disease, 61t
Propulsid (cisapride), 166
Prozac (fluoxetine), 68t, 157-158
Psychiatric disorders, 59t, 154-162, 155t
    levodopa-related, 159
    nursing home placement and, 159
    predisposing characteristics for, 158-159
    psychotherapy for, 181
    treatment of, 159-161
    triggering events for, 160
Psychogenic parkinsonism, 12t
Psychosis. See *Psychiatric disorders.*
Psychotherapy, 181
    family counseling and, 184-185
Pugilistic encephalopathy, 14-15
Pulmonary embolism, 21
Punch drunk boxer, 14-15
Putamen, 31, *32*
Pyramidal signs, in parkinsonism-plus syndromes vs Parkinson's
    disease, 65t
Pyridostigmine, 68t

Quality of life, 75t-76t, 83t, 169

Rating scales, from DATATOP, 19
Rating scales in Parkinson's disease, 72-73
    of complications of therapy, 80t-81t
    of daily living activities, 75t-76t, 83t
    of mentation, behavior, and mood, 72
    of motor function, 77t-79t
    Schwab and England Activities of Daily Living Scale as, 83t
    staging from, 81t
    Step-Second Test as, 82t
    Unified rating scale for parkinsonism as. See *Unified
Parkinson's Disease Rating Scale (UPDRS).*

Reglan (metoclopromide)
  contraindications to, 166
  indications for, 66
  parkinsonism from, 67t
Remacemide, 134-135
Requip. See *Ropinirole (Requip)*.
Reserpine, 12t, 14
  parkinsonism from, 66, 68t
Respiratory chain, 51
Resting tremor. See *Tremor, resting*.
Rigidity
  cogwheel, 11, 68
  in parkinsonism-plus syndromes vs Parkinson's disease, 65t
  physical therapy for, 178-180, 179t
  scale of, 77t
Rising from chair, rating of, 79t
Risperdal (risperidone), 67t
Ropinirole (Requip)
  action mechanism of, 110
  adjunctive, 112-115, *114*
  chemical structure of, 110
  dosage of, 92t, 115t, 115-116
  as monotherapy, 110-112, *112-113*
  pharmacokinetics of, 116
  selegiline effectiveness vs, 111, *113*
  side effects of, 112, 114-115, 159

Salivation, 75t, 183
Schwab and England Activities of Daily Living Scale, 83t, 107
Seborrheic dermatitis, 188-189
Secondary parkinsonism, 12t, 13-15
Selegiline (Eldepryl)
  adjunctive, 96, 99, *100*
  age and, 98
  cheese effect and, 98
  clinical studies of, 96-97
  cognitive impairment and, 98
  demerol interaction with, 183
  dosage of, 93t, 99
  indications for, *89*, 90
  as inhibitor of disease progression, 54
  monotherapy with, 98
  for MPTP intoxication, 27, 96
  as neuroprotectant, 96-98
  oxidative stress and, 98
  side effects of, 159-160
  SSRI interaction with, 158
  for wearing-off phenomenon, 149
Sensory changes, 59t
  rating of, 76t

12

Serentil (Mesoridazine), 67t
Serotonin uptake inhibitors, selective (SSRI), 157-158
Sertraline (Zoloft), 157
Serzone (nefazodone), 158
Sexuality, 189
Shy-Drager syndrome, 13t, 15
  components of, 64
  differential diagnosis of, 65t
Sialorrhea, 185, 187
  clozapine-induced, 161
Sinemet. See *Carbidopa/levodopa (Sinemet)*.
Single photon emission computed tomography (SPECT). See also
  Computed tomography (CT).
  in diagnosis of Parkinson's disease, 72
  in Parkinson's vs Alzheimer's dementia, 156
Skin
  levodopa-related pain in, 153
  seborrheic dermatitis of, 188-189
Sleep disorders, 59t
  rating scale of, 81t
  treatment of, 155t
  types of, 161-162
Smoking, 28
Sparine (Promazine), 67t
Spastic bulbar palsy (Binswanger's disease), 12t
  differential diagnosis of, 58, 62
Speech dysfunction, 75t
  scale of, 77t
Speech therapy, 180
SSRI (selective serotonin uptake inhibitor), 157-158
Staging of Parkinson's disease, 81t-83t
Stelazine (trifluoperazine), 67t
Step-Second Test, 82t
Striatonigral degeneration, 13t, 15
  in aging vs Parkinson's disease patient, 23-24, *25-26*
  differential diagnosis of, 58, 63, 65t
  iron in, 49-50
  levodopa for, 63
  in multiple system atrophy, 63
  positron emission tomography of, 71
  types of, 45
  wearing-off phenomenon and, 146-147, *147*
Striatum, 31, *32*
  in neurotransmitter balance, 36, *37*
Substantia nigra
  anatomy of, 31, *32*, 33
  environmental toxins and, 27
  levodopa toxicity and, 129
  normal, *33*

Substantia nigra (*continued*)
  oxidative stress and, 45-48
  in Parkinson's disease, 41, *42*, 45
  subregional divisions of, *25*
Subthalamic nucleus, 31, *32*, 134
Superoxide dismutase, chronic inhibition of, 49
Superoxide reduction, 45
Supine hypertension, 164
Support groups, 169
Supranuclear palsy, 15
  iron uptake and storage in, 50
  progressive, 13t
    differential diagnosis of, 58, 62-63, 65t
    glutathione levels in, 47
    positron emission tomography of, 71
Surgical management of Parkinson's disease, 9
  advances in, 191
  deep-brain stimulation in
    action mechanisms in, 204-205
    complications of, 201-202, 203t
    disadvantages of, 203
    effectiveness of, 200-201, *202*, 203-204
    patient selection for, 202
    techniques in, 199
  future directions in, 211-213
  gene therapy, autologous, 212
  gene transfer in, *in vivo*, 212
  immortalized cell implantation in, 213
  localization in, 191
  pallidotomy in
    advances in, 196
    basal ganglia circuitry and, *195*
    effectiveness of, 194, 196-197
    patient selection for, 197
  polymer-encapsulated dopamine-secreting cell implantation in, 211
  techniques in, 192-193, *193*, *195*
  thalamotomy in
    complications of, 198
    effectiveness of, 197-198
    history of, 197
    pallidotomy vs, 194
    patient selection for, 199
    techniques in, 192
  transplantation of dopamine-producing cells in
    donor tissues for, 205-206
    effectiveness of, 208, 209t, 210
    immunosuppression in, 207
    implantation site for, 206-207
    patient selection for, 207

12

Swallowing dysfunction (dysphasia), 59t, 75t
  treatment of, 185, 187
Swimming, 174
Symmetrel. See *Amantadine (Symmetrel)*.
α-Synuclein, 25
Syringomesencephalia, 12t

Taractan (chlorprothixene), 67t
Tasmar (tolcapone). See *Tolcapone (Tasmar)*.
Teamwork, therapeutic, 169-171
Tetrabenazine, 12t, 68t
Thalamic dementia syndrome, 13t
Thalamotomy
  complications of, 198
  effectiveness of, 197-198
  history of, 197
  pallidotomy vs, 194
  patient selection for, 199
  techniques in, 192
Thalamus, intralaminar nuclei of, 31, *32*, 33
Thienobenzodiazepine, 67t
Thiethylperazine (Norzine, Torecan), 67t
Thioridazine (Mellaril), 67t
Thiothixene (Navane), 67t
Thioxantheses, 67t
Thorazine (chlorpromazine), 67t
Thought disorders, 74t
α-Tocopherol. See *Vitamin E*.
Toe, dystonia of, 59t
Tolcapone (Tasmar). See also *Catechol-O-methyltransferase
    (COMT) inhibitors*.
  dosage of, 93t, 117, 120, 126t
  as early therapy, 119-120
  effectiveness of, *118*, 119, *121*
  as levodopa adjunct, 116-119, *118*
  pharmacokinetics of, 126t
  side effects of, 118, 120, 126t
  wearing-off phenomenon and, 119
Torecan (thiethylperazine), 67t
Toxin exposure, parkinsonism after, 12t
Transferrin, iron binding by, 46, 49
Transplantation of dopamine-producing cells. See *Dopamine-
    producing cell transplantation*.
TRAP, 11, 13
Trauma, parkinsonism after, 12t, 14-15
Trazodone, 157-158
Treatment of Parkinson's disease. See also *Complications of
    Parkinson's disease and treatment*.
  algorithm for, *89*

Treatment of Parkinson's disease. (*continued*)
  complications in, rating scales of, 80t-81t
  dental care in, 182-184
  discussion topics in, timetable for, 169, 170t
  driving in, 173
  family counseling in, 184-185
  in future, 9
  genetic, 9, 212-213
  home environmental modifications in, 171-173
  neuroprotective, 9, 87, 96-98, 135
  nonpharmacologic, 169-189
  occupational therapy in, 171-173, 181, 182t
  patient education in, 173-174, 174t
  pharmacologic. See *Drug therapy for Parkinson's disease.*
  physical therapy in, 174-175, *175-177*, 178-180, 179t
  psychotherapy in, 181
  quality of life in, 169
  restorative, 87. See also *Surgical management of Parkinson's disease.*
  speech therapy in, 180
  support groups in, 169
  surgical. See *Surgical management of Parkinson's disease.*
  symptomatic, 87
  team effort in, 169-171
  vitamin E in, 99-101
Tremor
  in classification of disease, 20-21
  essential, 50, 58, *60*, 61t
    age and, 60, 61t
    drawing by patient with, *60*
    treatment of, 61t
    vs Parkinson's disease, 58, 60, *60*, 61t
  familial, 24
  of hands, 77t
  internal, 141
  in parkinsonism-plus syndromes vs Parkinson's disease, 65t
  physical therapy for, 178-180, 179t
  pill-rolling, 68
  rating scale of, 76t
  resting, 11, 13, 57, 59t
    rating scale of, 77t
Tremor dominant disease, 20-21
Triavil (perphenazine and amitriptyline), 67t
Tricyclic antidepressants, 155t, 157
Trifluoperazine (Stelazine), 67t
Trihexyphenidyl (Artane), 91t, 94
Trilafon (perphenazine), 67t

12

Tumor
  dopamine-producing cells in, transplantation of. See
    Dopamine-producing cell transplantation.
  parkinsonism and, 12t
Twin studies, 24

Unified Parkinson's Disease Rating Scale (UPDRS), 74t-81t, 97
  after pallidotomy, 196
  pramipexole effectiveness on, 105-107, 109
  ropinirole effectiveness on, 110-112, *112-113*
Upper extremities
  changes in, 59t
  dexterity of, rating scales of, 78t
  in Parkinson's disease vs essential tremor, 61t
  tremor in, 77t
Urinary dysfunction, 154

Vascular parkinsonism, 12t
Venlafaxine (Effexor), 157
Vincristine (Oncovin), 68t
Visual hallucinations, 87, 154, 159. See also *Hallucinations.*
Vitamin E
  disease development/progression and, 129
  in early-onset disease, 99-101
  as free radical scavenger, 46-47
Vocalizations, nocturnal, 154, 155t, 161-162
von Economo's encephalitis, 13-14

Walking. See also *Gait.*
  as physical therapy, 174
Wearing-off phenomenon. See also *Dyskinesia.*
  entacapone and, 125
  pramipexole and, 106-107
  striatonigral degeneration and, 146-147, *147*
  symptoms of, 147-148
  timing of, *147*, 147-148
  tolcapone and, 119
  treatment of, 146t, 148-149
Western equine encephalitis, 14
Wilson's disease, 13t, 15, 17

Xerostomia, 75t, 183

Zoloft (sertraline), 157
Zyprexa (olanzapine), 67t, 155t, 161